THE

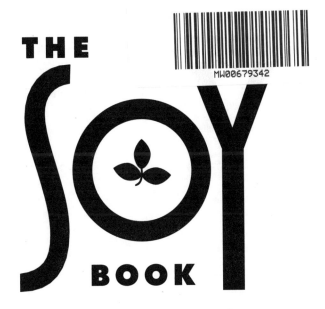

SOY
BOOK

ERIKA DILLMAN

WARNER BOOKS

A Time Warner Company

PUBLISHER'S NOTE: Neither this diet nor any other program should be followed without first consulting a health care professional. If you have any special conditions requiring attention, you should consult with your health care professional regularly regarding possible modification of the program contained in this book.

Copyright © 2001 by Erika Dillman
All rights reserved.

Warner Books, Inc., 1271 Avenue of the Americas, New York, NY 10020
Visit our Web site at www.twbookmark.com

 A Time Warner Company

Printed in the United States of America
First Printing: April 2001
10 9 8 7 6 5 4 3 2 1

Library of Congress Cataloging-in-Publication Data

Dillman, Erika.
    The little soy book / Erika Dillman.
        p. cm.
    Includes index.
    ISBN 0-446-67627-6
    1. Soyfoods—Health aspects. 2. Cookery (Soybeans) I. Title.

    RM666.S59 .D55 2001
    613.2'6—dc21   00-043864

Book design and text composition by L&G McRee
Cover design by Rachel McClain

Acknowledgments

I would like to thank the following people for their contributions to *The Little Soy Book:*

My agent, Anne Depue, and my editors, Diana Baroni and Molly Chehak, for their support and patience during the writing of this book.

All of the doctors, professors, researchers, and soy experts I spoke with during my research, for sharing their time and knowledge with me: Mark Messina, Ph.D.; Tom Clarkson, D.V.M., Professor of Comparative Medicine, Wake Forest University School of Medicine; Margo Woods, Ph.D., Associate Professor, Department of Family Medicine and Community Health, Tufts University School of Medicine; Brad Cortright, M.S., Research Specialist in Agriculture, National Soybean Re-

Acknowledgments

search Laboratory, University of Illinois; Maurice Bennink, Ph.D., Professor of Nutrition, Michigan State University; Tammy J. Stephenson, Ph.D. candidate, Department of Nutritional Sciences, University of Kentucky; Bill Shurtleff; Jin-Rong Zhou, Ph.D., Director of the Nutrition Metabolism Laboratory, Beth Israel Deaconess Medical Center, and Professor of Surgery, Harvard Medical Center; Mindy Kurzer, Ph.D., Associate Professor, University of Minnesota; Omer Kucuk, M.D., Professor of Medicine, Karmanos Cancer Institute, Wayne State University; Paula Boggs, North American Menopause Society; Georgina W. Sikorski, Protein Technologies International; the Alabama Department of Health, and the staffs of the Indiana Soy Board, the Ohio Soy Board, and the United Soy Board. And a very special thanks to Stephen Barnes, Ph.D., Professor of Pharmacology and Toxicology, and Helen Kim, Ph.D., Research Associate Professor, Department of Pharmacology and Toxicology, both of the University of Alabama-Birmingham.

Gail Simon, who created all of the wonderful recipes in this book, and Tiana Colvolos of Pacific Northwest Nutrition Services, for providing nutrition information about soy.

Terence Pagard, for proofreading, and Caitlin Dundon, for helping me when my computer refused to cooperate.

Acknowledgments

Leah Ankeny and Laurie Bohm, for taste testing the soy recipes.

Patti McCall, Cindy Mitchell, Elena Larkin, and the rest of the staff at Queen Anne Avenue Books; the members of my writing group, Ted Johnson, Suzan Huney, Jill Irwin, and Norman Glassman; and my friends and family for their support and encouragement.

Contents

Introduction

Growing up in rural Illinois, I was literally surrounded by the soybeans and corn that grew in the fields near my house. I thought that soybeans were only fed to cows and pigs, so when I was eight years old and was served a soy burger at school, I eyed it suspiciously, took one bite, and then let it slide off my plastic lunch tray into the garbage. It wasn't thick and juicy like the hamburgers my mother made, and it didn't taste like a McDonald's hamburger. From that day on, I brought peanut butter sandwiches on hamburger day.

My next encounter with soy occurred when I was fourteen years old and working for an agriculture company, detasseling corn. Most days we worked in the cornfields from 6 A.M. until late in the afternoon. Some days we walked beans, which involved walking up and down rows of soybean plants with a shovel, killing any threatening weeds or rogue corn stalks that we found. I always preferred walking beans because it was much easier work than trying to detassel miles-long rows of corn that were two feet taller than I was. My editor, who has lived in New York City all her life, finds it hilarious that I spent my summer vacations this way and that I continued to work in the fields for seven straight summers. I think it was a portent.

I finally discovered tofu in college when some friends added it to a vegetable stir-fry at a dinner party I was attending. I didn't really know what it was or what to do with it, but I liked its texture and how it soaked up all the flavors of the garlic, vegetables, and sauce with which it was cooked. In the years since that dinner party, tofu has become an important protein source for me as part of my vegetarian diet.

More recently, I've incorporated many other soy foods into my meals, including roasted soy nuts, tempeh, soy sausages, soy-based nutrition bars, and miso soup. I have to admit that I was surprised that I liked so many of them. The first time I ate a soy breakfast sausage I was amazed that it had the same taste, texture, and smell as the pork sausages I had eaten as a child. I had to double-check the ingredients on the box to make sure I wasn't eating meat.

This book is for people who may be uninformed about soy foods, as I was, or simply curious about soy's health benefits. Eating soy has helped me create more variety in my diet while helping me get the protein I need. I hope you will enjoy learning about all the different types of soy foods as much as I have.

Enjoy.

ERIKA DILLMAN

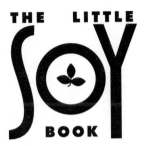

THE LITTLE

SOY

BOOK

1 It's Soy Time

The modest little soybean has hit the big time. You can't open a magazine or a newspaper these days without seeing an article about soy. Veggie burgers containing soy are selling like hotcakes. Tofu, made from soybeans, is now widely available in supermarkets across the country. You can even get soy milk lattes at Starbucks.

So what's all the fuss about? Americans are starting to realize what Asians have known for thousands of years: soybeans pack a huge nutritional punch. High in protein and low in fat, they're an inexpensive, fiber-rich, cholesterol-free food. Soy also contains powerful plant chemicals called isoflavones that researchers believe show potential for fighting many chronic diseases. Most notably, soy has been shown to help fight heart disease by lowering cholesterol, a claim approved by the U.S. Food and Drug Administration (FDA).

For people trying to reduce their fat and cholesterol intake, and for vegetarians looking for a high-quality protein source, soy is the ideal food—easy to cook with and available in a variety of styles and products.

In *The Little Soy Book* you'll learn about soy's nutritional qualities and health benefits, the role isoflavones play in fighting disease, the many different types of soy foods and how to incorporate them into your diet, and finally, how to cook with soy. In the final chapter you'll find thirty recipes.

But first, a brief introduction to the humble bean.

WHAT'S A SOYBEAN?

Soybeans are small, green, oval-shaped legumes that grow in pods, like peas, on the soybean plant. The beans are harvested about four months after they're planted, when they have become hard, dry, and yellow. There are also brown and black varieties of soybeans.

Soy Uses

Soy has been called "the wonder bean" and "a miracle crop," and it's no surprise. Every bit of the bean has a use. Whole soybeans can be fermented, curdled, and pressed to make traditional soy foods like soy sauce, tofu, and soy milk. Soy can also be processed to create a wide range of food and agricultural products. First the hulls (outer shell of the bean) are removed and processed to make livestock feed and fiber additives for food products like packaged bread and cereal. Once the hulls are removed, the beans are rolled into flakes from which soy oil is extracted. The flakes are then made into livestock feed, or they are further processed to make a variety of soy protein products like flour, soy milk, soup mixes, and other foods. Soy oil is also refined and used in food products as well as industrial products.

Here are just a few products that contain soy:

Agriculture/Industry: Livestock feed, pet food, pesticides/fungicides, cleaners, paint, ink, plastics, adhesives, dust-control agents, biodiesel fuel, disinfectants, epoxies, polyesters, textiles, crayons, cosmetics, candles, hair conditioner and other hair-styling products.

Foods: Cooking oil, margarine, mayonnaise, soy milk, meat substitutes, baby food and infant formula, flour, ice cream, roasted soy nuts, cereals, tofu, miso, tempeh.

The United States produces half of the world's soybeans, and U.S. soybean and soy product exports generated more than $7 billion in 1998.

HISTORY OF SOY

Soybeans were first cultivated from wild plants by Chinese farmers five thousand years ago. According to ancient texts, soybeans were used as both a food and a medicine and were one of five designated "sacred" crops. Over time, soybeans were also grown in southeast Asia, Korea, and Japan. Today soy remains a staple food in many Asian countries. The average Japanese person eats more than fifty pounds of tofu a year, and until recently, soy milk was more popular in China than Coca-Cola.

It's Soy Time

It wasn't until the early 1800s that soybeans were introduced to Europe and America. Soybeans were most likely brought to Europe by traders who carried them back from China. Soybeans arrived in America during this time stored in barrels that were used as ballast in trading ships. Most of the beans were thrown out when the ships arrived, but a few farmers began experimenting with the seeds. Benjamin Franklin was one of America's first soy enthusiasts, sending soybean seeds to America from France after learning about Chinese tofu.

By the late 1800s American farmers were growing soybeans for cattle feed, and in 1904 George Washington Carver discovered that soybeans were a great source of protein and oil.

In the beginning of the twentieth century, American scientists began to study thousands of soybean varieties from China. At that time, America imported 40 percent of its edible fats and oil, but when soybean fields in China were destroyed during World War II, the United States stepped up its soybean production.

Automobile manufacturer and vegetarian Henry Ford was a pioneer in soy research and soy promotion. In the 1930s he and his scientists experimented with making foods out of soy, including meat alternatives, milk, ice cream, and butter. He wore soy clothing (suits that were woven from a blend of wool and soy fibers) and even made a car out of soy plastic. In the 1960s and 1970s, it was Ford's scientists who worked with food manufacturers to incorporate soy into food products.

Today the United States is the largest producer and exporter of soybeans, which are grown in more than thirty states, with Iowa, Illinois, Minnesota, Indiana, Ohio, Missouri, and Nebraska among the top producers. In 1998, American soybean farmers produced a record-breaking 2,757 billion bushels of soybeans.

WORLD SOYBEAN PRODUCTION, 1998

48 percent	United States
20 percent	Brazil
12 percent	Argentina
9 percent	China
3 percent	India
2 percent	Paraguay
1 percent	Europe
5 percent	Other

(Source: *Soy Stats 1999*)

Soy Foods

You've probably used soy sauce before, and heard of tofu and soy milk, but maybe you didn't know that soy comes in many different forms . . . or that you probably have eaten soy many times without knowing it. Widely used by food manufacturers, soy and soy products are common ingredients in packaged foods such as candy bars, powdered soup mixes, cereals, and baby food. Most of the vegetable oil you'll find at the grocery store is actually 100 percent soybean oil.

Soy, in the form of TSP (textured soy protein, also called textured vegetable protein or TVP), has been used for years in ground meat as an extender and to add texture. Low in fat and high in protein, soy is also used to make low-fat margarine, nutrition bars, and protein powder used in smoothies, thick shake-like drinks containing ingredients like fruit, water, soy milk or yogurt, and nutritional supplements.

This book will help you learn about the many types of soy foods and how to add them to your diet, why soy is becoming such a popular food, and how you can gain important health benefits from eating soy.

2 Why Eat Soy?

Forget about the soy you knew in the seventies; the new soy is delicious, versatile, and fun to eat. Soy-processing technology has significantly improved in the past thirty years, resulting in many great-tasting soy-based foods, and as Asian dishes have become more popular in this country, food manufacturers are spicing up some traditional soy foods like tofu and tempeh to be more appealing to a Western palate. From hickory-smoked tofu chunks to BBQ tempeh to raspberry soy yogurt, a wide array of soy products is available.

Eating soy is an excellent way to add variety to your diet and to gain many important health benefits, like reducing your fat and cholesterol intake. A rich source of nutrients, vitamins, minerals, and high-quality protein, soy is the perfect addition to a low-fat diet and a valuable substitute for higher-fat foods like meat and dairy. For millions of Americans trying to cut the fat in their diets, soy can help.

SOY PACKS A PUNCH

Nutritionally, soy has an impressive résumé. In addition to the high-quality protein it provides, soy is a low-fat, cholesterol-free food. It's also a great source of essential nutrients such as calcium, iron, zinc, vitamin B_6, thiamin, riboflavin, niacin, folate, phosphorus, potassium, and fiber. Soy contains omega-3 fatty acids that are similar to the beneficial fatty acids found in fish, and linoleic acid, another essential fat. Both of these fatty acids have been shown to be beneficial to heart health.

WHAT'S IN A BEAN

Soy contains

38 percent protein
18 percent oil
15 percent soluble carbohydrates
15 percent insoluble carbohydrates (fiber)
14 percent water, ash, other

(Source: United Soybean Board)

NUTRITIONAL CONTENT OF SOY FOODS

The following chart describes some of the main soy foods and their nutritional values. Figures have been rounded to the nearest whole number.

As you can see, all soy foods are not the same. The different processes used to make these foods result in products with varied nutritional profiles, and values will vary from brand to brand. For example, tofu is a great source of calcium and very

Why Eat Soy?

---

low in sodium. Soy sauces, on the other hand, do not provide significant amounts of calcium and are very high in sodium. You will also notice that across the board, soy is low in fat. Even the higher-fat foods like roasted soybeans and soy flour contain more polyunsaturated fat than saturated fat.

Soy food	Serving size	Calories (kcal)	Protein (g)	Fat (g)	Carbo—hydrate (g)	Fiber (g)	Calcium (mg)	Iron (mg)	Zinc (mg)	Sodium (mg)
Miso	½ c	206	12	6	28	3	66	3	3	3,647
Tofu, raw, firm	½ c	145	16	9	4	0	205	10	2	14
Tofu, raw, regular	½ c	76	8	5	2	0	105	5	1	7
Soybeans, cooked, boiled	½ c	173	17	9	10	2	102	5	1	1
Soybeans, dry roasted	½ c	450	40	22	33	5	270	4	5	2
Soybeans, raw	½ c	416	37	20	30	5	277	16	5	2
Soybeans, roasted	½ c	474	35	25	34	5	138	4	3	163
Soy milk	½ c	33	3	2	2	1	4	1	0	12
Tempeh	½ c	199	19	8	17	3	93	2	2	6
Soy flour, defatted, stirred	½ c	329	47	1	38	4	241	9	2	20

Soy food	Serving size	Calories (kcal)	Protein (g)	Fat (g)	Carbo‑hydrate (g)	Fiber (g)	Calcium (mg)	Iron (mg)	Zinc (mg)	Sodium (mg)
Soy flour, full-fat, raw, stirred	½ c	436	35	21	35	5	206	6	4	13
Soy flour, full-fat, roasted, stirred	½ c	441	35	22	34	2	188	6	4	12
Soy flour, low-fat, stirred	½ c	326	47	7	38	4	188	6	1	18
Soy protein isolate	1 oz.	338	81	3	7	0	178	15	4	1,005
Soy sauce made from soy and wheat (shoyu)	1 T	53	5	0	9	0	17	2	0	5,715
Soy sauce made from soy only (tamari)	1 T	60	11	0	6	0	20	2	0	5,586
Soy sauce made from HVP (hydrolyzed vegetable protein)	1 T	41	2	0	8	0	5	1	0	5,690
Natto	½ c	212	18	11	14	2	217	9	3	7
Okara	½ c	77	3	2	13	4	80	1	n/a	9

(Source: *1999 U.S. Soyfoods Directory*)

Why Eat Soy?

PERFECT PROTEIN

Whether you would like to reduce your intake of saturated fat and cholesterol or you're a vegetarian looking for a high-quality protein source, soy can help you meet your protein needs.

When you eat protein, it's broken down in your body into amino acids, which are then remade into the proteins your body needs. Unlike other plant foods, soy contains all nine essential amino acids, which makes it a high-quality protein that is virtually equal to animal protein. Your body naturally produces eleven of the twenty amino acids; the rest come from the foods you eat. If your meals also contain the recommended amounts of fruits, vegetables, and grains, your protein and other nutrient requirements will easily be met by incorporating soy into your diet.

Not only does soy provide high-quality protein, it is equal to animal protein in digestibility. Soy foods that have been cooked, heated, or fermented, like tofu and tempeh, are the most digestible.

What makes soy such an ideal source of protein is that, unlike meat or cheese, soy is cholesterol-free and low in fat. As you can see in the chart on page 11, only one-half cup of tofu provides 16 grams of protein and one-half cup of roasted soy nuts provides 40 grams of protein. Compared to beef, pork, or chicken, soy provides plenty of protein without the saturated fat or cholesterol found in animal products. For example, a 100-gram serving of hamburger provides 24 grams of protein, but 7.5 grams of saturated fat and 84 milligrams of cholesterol. A veggie burger made with soy provides 20 grams of protein, with only 1 gram of saturated fat and no cholesterol.

The chart on the following page shows how replacing some meats with soy meat alternatives can help you reduce your fat, cholesterol, and caloric intake. In addition to the soy products listed here, there are many other meat alternatives available including ground round, vegetable patties, Canadian bacon, deli slices like soy-based turkey and ham, and pepperoni, all made from soy.

Ta-tou is the Chinese word for soybean;
it means "greater bean."

Why Eat Soy?

Product	Serving size (g)	Calories	Total fat (g)	Saturated fat (g)	Choles-terol (mg)	Sodium (mg)	Protein (g)
Oscar Mayer Beef Bologna	1 slice (28 g)	90	8	4	15	300	3
Lightlife Smart Deli Bologna (soy)	3 slices (43 g)	50	0	0	0	300	10
Oscar Mayer Beef Franks	1 link (45 g)	140	13	6	30	460	5
Yves Tofu Wieners (soy)	1 link (38 g)	47	0.4	0	0	241	9
Italian sausage (pork)	75 g	242	21.5	7.8	25	465	12
Lightlife Italian sausage (soy)	1 link (40 g)	60	2	1	0	160	5
Hatfield Breakfast Links	3 links (59 g)	200	16	7	40	640	12
Yves Veggie Breakfast Links (soy)	2 links (50 g)	65	0	0	0	364	12
Oscar Mayer Smoked Cook Ham	3 slices (63 g)	60	2.5	1	30	750	10
Lightlife Smart Deli Ham (soy)	3 slices (43 g)	50	0	0	0	300	10

CUT THE FAT

When trying to reduce your fat intake, it's important to understand the different types of fat, which are defined by their saturation or solidity. The higher the saturation, the more harmful the fat is to your body. Saturated fats, found in animal protein like meat and cheese, remain solid at room temperature. They also promote cholesterol production in the body and clog arteries, increasing heart-disease risk. Polyunsaturated fats, found in sunflower, safflower, and soybean oil, are healthier than saturated fats. Unfortunately, when polyunsaturated fats are chemically altered to make other products like margarine, they are just as unhealthy as saturated fats. Monounsaturated fats are the healthiest fats because they do not increase cholesterol levels. Sources of monounsaturated fats include olives, avocados, and some nuts.

Eating soy in place of higher-fat foods is one way of lowering overall fat and cholesterol intake. The chart on the following page shows how many calories, fat grams, and cholesterol milligrams are saved by replacing some common meat and dairy products with soy foods.

Foods	Soy food substitution	Serving size	Fat grams saved	Cholesterol milligrams saved	Calories saved
Ground beef (85% lean)	½ cup textured vegetable protein granules, rehydrated (regular or beef flavored)	3-ounce portion, cooked	14	71	99
Chicken breast (skinned and cubed in small chunks)	½ cup textured vegetable protein chunks, rehydrated (chicken flavored)	3-ounce portion, cooked	3	77	58
Egg (as leavening agent in baking)	¼ cup silken "lite" firm tofu, mashed	Equivalent to one egg	4.5	213	53
Cheddar cheese	Soy-based cheddar cheese	1 ounce	4	30	36
Ricotta cheese (part skim)	Firm tofu, mashed	1 tablespoon	0	5	0
Whole milk	Regular soy milk or regular soy milk made from soy milk powder	8 ounces	4	33	70
2% milk	Reduced-fat soy milk or reduced-fat soy milk made from soy milk powder	8 ounces	3	18	20
Sour cream	Tofu sour cream	1 tablespoon	2.5	5	19

(Source: *1999 U.S. Soyfoods Directory*)

HOW MUCH PROTEIN DO YOU NEED?

To determine your daily protein requirements, multiply your weight by .364

Weight in lbs. × .364 = ___ grams/day.

Example: A 130-pound (59-kilogram) woman needs 47 grams of protein per day.

SOY AND HEALTH

As researchers and doctors learn more about the role diet plays in health and disease, health organizations like the American Heart Association and the American Cancer Society are recommending diets that are low in saturated fat and cholesterol.

Americans love their meat, cheese, and eggs. They also mistakenly believe that they need to be concerned with getting enough protein in their diets. The fact is, Americans eat plenty of protein, but often too much of it comes from animal products, which are high in fat and cholesterol.

If you compare the typical Western diet with the typical Asian diet, which consists of vegetables, grains, and soy foods, it's no wonder that the populations in countries where the Asian diet is typical have lower rates of heart disease and some types of cancer.

Doctors, researchers, health organizations, and even government agencies agree that the old food pyramid needs revising, and over the past decade there have been changes. One significant change is the recommendation to increase consumption of fruits and vegetables from a few servings a day to nine or ten servings a day.

The American Institute for Cancer Research goes further in advocating changes in the U.S. Dietary Guidelines. They recommend diets that

- Place plant-based foods in the center of every meal
- Contain a variety of foods (and foods that have minimal processing)
- Are based on whole foods (and that do not rely on nutritional supplements for disease prevention)
- Are free from excessive amounts of added sugar, salt, and fat

Replacing animal protein in the diet with plant protein is one way to lower your intake of saturated fat and cholesterol, reduce your overall calorie intake, and increase your fiber intake.

THE FOOD PYRAMID

Based on the dietary guidelines developed by the U.S. Department of Agriculture, the Food Pyramid outlines the five major food groups from which you should eat each day in order to fulfill your body's nutritional requirements. The chart below describes the daily servings you need to eat from each group.

Food groups in pyramid	Recommended daily servings	Examples of serving sizes, including soy foods
Bread, cereal, rice, and pasta	6–11 servings	1 slice bread; 1 oz. breakfast cereal; ½ C pasta, rice, or cooked cereal; ½ C soy grits
Fruit	2–4 servings	1 medium orange, apple, or banana; ¾ C fruit juice; ½ C chopped or canned fruit

Why Eat Soy?

Food groups in pyramid	Recommended daily servings	Examples of serving sizes, including soy foods
Vegetables	3–5 servings	1 c raw leafy vegetables; ½ c cooked (or raw chopped) vegetables; ¾ c vegetable juice
Meat, poultry, fish, beans, eggs, and nuts	2–3 servings	2–3 oz. cooked lean meat, poultry, or fish; ½ c dry beans; 1 egg; 2 T peanut butter; 3 oz. tofu; ½ c cooked soybeans
Milk, yogurt, and cheese	2–3 servings	1 c milk or yogurt; 1½ oz. cheese; 1 c soy milk or soy yogurt; 2 oz. soy cheese
Fats, oils, and sweets	Use sparingly	

(Sources: U.S. Department of Agriculture; Ohio Soybean Council)

Substituting soy foods for some of the foods in the pyramid is one way to lower your fat and cholesterol intake while still gaining important nutrients. Soy flour can replace some of the flour in baked goods to boost their protein content, and soybeans can fill in for foods in the meat group (one-half cup of cooked soybeans is equal to one ounce of meat, and a three-ounce soy-based veggie patty counts as one serving of meat). There are even soy alternatives for the dairy group: one cup of soy yogurt equals one serving of dairy. Finally, using soybean oil is a great choice for the fats group; it's low in saturated fat and high in polyunsaturated fat. While you should use fats sparingly, remember that fat is necessary in the diet and shouldn't be eliminated entirely. It helps transport fat-soluble vitamins throughout the body.

SOY AND CHOLESTEROL

As many of us know, high cholesterol increases heart-disease risk. Researchers have been studying soy's potential health benefits for more than thirty years, especially in the area of heart health. In more than fifty studies, soy protein was shown to lower total cholesterol and LDL cholesterol (the "bad cholesterol") in people with high cholesterol. LDL, which stands for low-density lipoprotein, delivers cholesterol to the body's tissues. It is often referred to as the bad cholesterol because it can accumulate in the bloodstream, causing damage to arteries and clogging the arteries, known as atherosclerosis. High LDL levels are associated with high heart-disease risk.

Why Eat Soy?

———

HDL, high-density lipoprotein (the "good cholesterol"), delivers cholesterol to the liver, where it is broken down and eliminated from the body. HDL is also believed to remove cholesterol from artery walls and prevent heart disease.

FDA APPROVAL

Based on the results of cholesterol studies mentioned on the previous page, the Food and Drug Administration ruled in 1999 that it would approve a health claim for products containing soy protein.

The FDA ruling allows food manufacturers to print on their labels that 25 grams of soy protein a day, as part of a diet low in saturated fat and cholesterol, may reduce the risk of heart disease. To carry this claim, foods must provide 6.25 grams of protein per serving (approximately one-fourth of the recommended daily amount) and contain no more than 1 gram of saturated fat, 3 grams of total fat, 20 milligrams of cholesterol, and 480 milligrams of sodium.

ADDING SOY TO YOUR DIET

Many people are reluctant to try soy foods because they think that they won't like them. They think of soy as a bland-tasting, boring food, even if they know about soy's stellar nutritional profile. It's very common to resist change, especially when it comes to food, but in soy's case, it's worth your while to give soy another look.

Soy has come a long way since the drab little soy-enhanced hamburgers many of us were served in school lunches in the seventies. The quality, taste, and texture of soy products used in foods have improved dramatically, and whole soy foods are more widely available to consumers at natural food stores and even supermarkets.

If you've ever eaten at a Chinese or Thai restaurant, you know how delicious tofu is when it's mixed in a basil-garlic stir-fry or deep-fried and served on a bed of spinach, smothered in peanut sauce.

It's easy to add soy to your diet. You can use soy milk in your cereal, sprinkle soy nuts on your breakfast yogurt or lunch salad, make a sandwich with soy deli meats and cheeses, add tofu and tempeh to your favorite vegetable dishes, and use soybeans in chili. In chapter 5 I've included more ideas and recipes to show you how easy and tasty it is to add soy to your diet.

WHAT'S A SERVING SIZE?

You don't have to eat a lot of soy to gain health benefits. Just one-half cup of many soy foods equals a serving size. For example, if you have one-fourth cup of soy nuts on your morning yogurt and then eat one-half cup of firm tofu in a stir-fry for dinner, you'll exceed the daily twenty-five grams of soy protein recommended by the FDA to gain heart-health benefits.

Each of these measurements is equal to one serving of soy food:

1 cup of soy milk
½ cup of tofu
½ cup of tempeh
½ cup of cooked soybeans
½ cup of edamame beans
½ cup of textured soy protein (rehydrated)
¼ cup of defatted soy flour
¼ cup of soy nuts
2 tablespoons of miso

(Source: *1999 U.S. Soyfoods Directory*)

BENEFITS OF EATING SOY

Here are a few good reasons to consider soy:

- Eating soy foods is a great way to lower your intake of saturated (and total) fat, cholesterol, and calories.
- Soy protein lowers cholesterol in people with high cholesterol when part of a low-fat, low-cholesterol diet.
- Soy is a nutritional powerhouse and a perfect substitute for animal protein.
- Soy cheese, soy ice cream, and other soy dairy products are great alternatives for people who are lactose intolerant or want to enjoy "dairy" treats without the guilt.
- Soy comes in many different forms; you can eat it for breakfast, lunch, and dinner.
- Vegetarians can join in the fun at cookouts! When everyone throws their burgers on the grill, you can grill a veggie burger, a soy chicken breast, or better yet, a delicious soy Italian sausage.

How Much Soy Is Enough?

While the FDA guidelines recommend twenty-five grams of soy protein a day for cholesterol-lowering benefits, there are no established guidelines about how much soy a person needs to eat to gain other health benefits. It's probably more helpful to think of soy in serving sizes and as a protein substitute for high-fat, high-cholesterol foods.

For example, if you look at the servings chart on page 11, you'll see that it takes only one-half cup of tofu, soybeans, or tempeh to equal one serving size. On the same chart you'll see that just one-half cup of tempeh has nineteen grams of protein; that's almost half the daily requirements for the 130-pound woman described in the example. And it nearly meets the twenty-five grams necessary for cholesterol-lowering benefits.

Which Soy Foods Are Best

After reading about the FDA ruling and hearing other soy health claims in the news, you might be wondering which soy foods to eat. As with many other foods, the general rule applies—it's always best to eat whole foods and limit the amount of processed foods you eat. Soybeans, tofu, tempeh, miso, and soy nuts are all made using the whole soybean and therefore provide a rich and natural source of protein and other nutrients. As you'll notice on the chart on page 11, the amount of nutrients varies from food to food.

For people who are reluctant to eat soy foods, soy protein isolate, which contains 70 percent protein and is a common ingredient in protein drink powders and nutrition bars, can be a first introduction to soy. While soy protein isolate provides a significant serving of protein, it is the most processed soy food. When soybeans are processed to make this substance, they are washed either with water or with alcohol. Unfortunately, the alcohol washes away some of the important elements of the soy, namely the isoflavones, which are plant compounds thought to have beneficial properties (isoflavones and their potential to fight disease will be discussed in the next chapter).

Faced with the variety of soy foods and soy products out there, you may want to consider how different products are prepared. Because this type of information is rarely printed on food labels, you may decide to stick with whole soy foods.

3 Health Benefits of Soy

There's no doubt that soy is a nutrition-packed food and that it's a great addition to a healthy diet. The question is, can soy help prevent and treat disease?

Soy has been touted in the media, and by some food and soy-supplement manufacturers, as a superfood that may ward off heart disease and cancer as well as reduce menopausal symptoms and prevent bone loss from osteoporosis.

According to research completed to date, soy's potential to fight disease looks promising. Soy protein, as part of a low-fat diet, has been shown to lower cholesterol in people with high cholesterol, and soy isoflavones, a type of plant chemical highly concentrated in soy, may help prevent or delay some disease processes.

This chapter provides an overview of soy's potential for helping fight chronic diseases and other health concerns, as well as an explanation of soy isoflavones and their role in fighting disease. (Please keep in mind that this book is not meant to be a scientific or medical journal, just a guide to help you learn more about soy foods and some of the issues involved with soy research.)

SOY AND DIET

A good place to start when talking about soy research is a comparison between the Asian diet and the Western diet. The average Asian diet is low in animal protein and high in plant protein, including soy foods. The Western diet, on the other hand, is characterized by high consumption of animal protein and foods high in cholesterol and saturated fat.

Studies have shown that in countries where the Asian diet is typical, rates of heart disease, breast cancer, colon cancer, and prostate cancer are lower than in the United States. Japan is a perfect example of this phenomenon. It has a low rate of hormone-dependent cancer (that is, cancer that requires hormones to develop) and one-fourth the mortality rate from breast cancer and prostate cancer of the United States.

Researchers have also discovered that Asians who move to the United States and adopt a traditional Western diet eventually have the same rates of breast and prostate cancer as Americans. This leads them to believe that diet plays some role in fighting disease. In fact, the National Cancer Institute estimates that 30 percent of cancer is diet related. Researchers are now focusing on studying foods like soy, which may protect health and promote healing.

SOY ISOFLAVONES

If you have heard about soy's health benefits, you've probably also heard about isoflavones.

Every plant contains phytochemicals, compounds of plant chemicals that have no nutritional (or caloric) value but are physiologically active in the body. Soybeans contain many different phytochemicals, including a type called isoflavones, which are more highly concentrated in soy than in other plants.

Isoflavones are complex substances that function in a variety of ways. They have a chemical structure similar to the hormone estrogen, although they are much weaker than the body's naturally produced estrogen. Sometimes isoflavones work in the body like estrogen, and sometimes they work as "antiestrogens," interfering with or blocking the body's normal estrogen function. The complexity of isoflavones makes it difficult for researchers to reach conclusive, consistent results concerning soy isoflavones in relation to human health.

How Soy Fights Disease

Researchers have been studying soy isoflavones for many years to determine how they function in the body. One type of isoflavone, called genistein, has been the subject of much soy research. Laboratory studies have shown that genistein may halt the growth and proliferation of cancer cells, prevent the formation of blood vessels that feed cancerous tumors, and work as an antioxidant, preventing the formation of oxygen-free radicals, highly reactive molecules that damage healthy cells. What researchers still don't know is how some of the isoflavones work on the body, or whether the isoflavones work best alone or in combination with soy protein.

In addition to isoflavones, soy contains five known cancer-fighting substances, called anticarcinogens (these substances are also found in other plants): protease inhibitors, which interfere with the enzymes that promote tumor growth; phytate, an antioxidant that inhibits cancer growth; phytoterols, which chemically resemble cholesterol and have been shown to lower blood cholesterol levels; saponins, antioxidants that also resemble cholesterol and help reduce blood cholesterol; and phenolic acid, an antioxidant that halts the formation of some cancer-causing agents. Soy also contains fiber, which helps reduce cholesterol; lecithin, which may also help reduce cholesterol; and omega-3 fatty acids, which are believed to help lower the risk of heart disease.

Soy Research

Much of soy research has been focused on looking at how soy protein and soy isoflavones work in the body to determine if and how they promote health and fight disease. There are no clear-cut answers yet, but as you will read in the following pages, many studies have shown positive results.

Some of the questions researchers are trying to answer include the following:

- Do isoflavones have the potential to fight cancer and other diseases in humans?
- How do isoflavones work?
- What is the relationship between soy protein and isoflavones in fighting disease? Are they more beneficial in combination or separately?
- What amount of isoflavones and/or soy protein provides helpful effects?
- What amount of isoflavones and/or soy protein may produce harmful effects?
- Which soy foods are the best sources of isoflavones and protein?
- How do soy's anticarcinogenic substances work in the body?

Most of the research to date, which you may have read or

heard about in the media, has been epidemiological, in vitro, or in vivo (primarily using animal models). Although many human studies have been done, the true tests of the theories about soy have not been carried out in large-scale, long-term, well-controlled human studies simply because it has only been in the last decade that the active compounds in soy, isoflavones, have been identified.

You may have heard about soy research in the news and wondered about what some of these studies mean for your health, especially when the results sound negative. Two studies in particular have raised questions for consumers. One study suggested that soy may have an adverse effect on the thyroid, and another reported that high tofu intake was associated with cognitive impairment and even Alzheimer's disease. Some of the top U.S. researchers have pointed out that it's important to realize how studies are conducted and also that one study is not enough to allow conclusions. For example, the thyroid study was done using mice that were fed massive amounts of soy. Animal results do not always extrapolate to human health. In human populations that consume a lot of soy, there has been no significant incidence of thyroid disease.

The same can be said about the brain study. The study was

not conducted in a way that would allow researchers to establish true cause and effect, and controlled laboratory studies contradict the finding linking high tofu consumption with increased cognitive impairment. In other words, until more studies on these subjects can be completed, the results are preliminary and researchers feel that there is no reason for concern. Soy is safe to eat and provides many important health benefits.

Soy and Disease

The following pages list some of the different health benefits of eating soy foods. Each section describes the primary health benefit, gives a brief explanation of the disease, and mentions a few study results.

Heart Disease

Of all the health claims made about soy, its ability to fight heart disease by lowering cholesterol is the most widely accepted by researchers. Soy's cholesterol-lowering effects have been consistently demonstrated in dozens of studies around the world.

In fact, based on more than fifty of these studies, the FDA now allows soy manufacturers to print health claims on certain soy products. (See page 23 for more information about the FDA claim).

Too much cholesterol and saturated fat in the diet can increase blood cholesterol levels, which in turn increases the risk for atherosclerosis (i.e., clogged arteries), the primary risk factor for heart attacks and heart disease. According to the American Heart Association, heart disease is the leading cause of death for men and women in the United States, and more than one in four persons have some form of cardiovascular disease.

To prevent and treat heart disease, the American Heart Association recommends a low-fat, low-cholesterol, low-sodium diet. The goal behind a heart-healthy diet is to lower saturated fat intake, the total cholesterol count, and the level of LDL cholesterol (the "bad" cholesterol).

Studies have shown the following results:

- Replacing animal protein with soy protein in the diet lowered LDL cholesterol in people with high cholesterol.
- Soy lowered LDL cholesterol and triglycerides without lowering HDL (the "good" cholesterol).

- Soy lowered cholesterol and improved the ratio of HDL to LDL cholesterol.
- For people with very high cholesterol levels, soy lowered LDL cholesterol by 22 to 25 percent and lowered total cholesterol by up to 23 percent.

Other promising results:

- Soy protein may prevent cholesterol in the bloodstream from undergoing changes that make it damaging to artery walls.
- Genistein in test tubes halted the growth of plaque cells (plaque lines artery walls, increasing the risk of heart disease).
- Genistein may inhibit blood clot formation.
- Soy may help maintain a more desirable blood pressure.

Soy and Cancer

As with heart disease, lower rates of certain types of cancer in some Asian countries led researchers to believe that diet may play a role in disease prevention.

Cancer is the second leading cause of death in the United States. According to the American Cancer Society, one out of every four persons in the United States dies of cancer, and one out of every three will have cancer in his or her lifetime.

Studies have focused on the relationship between consuming soy foods and decreased cancer risk. The estrogenic effect of soy isoflavones has been a subject of study, particularly in the case of diseases that affect women like hormone-dependent cancers, osteoporosis, and heart disease, as well as health conditions like menopause. Other research has focused on the ability of isoflavones like genistein to slow or halt the growth of cancerous tumors.

Colon Cancer

Studies have shown that soy may help delay the onset of colon cancer and also have preventive effects.

Colon cancer is the third most common type of cancer in the United States. According to the American Cancer Society, 130,200 men and women will be diagnosed with colorectal cancers this year and 56,300 will die of it.

Colon cancer is another disease that doctors believe is influenced by diet. The American Cancer Society (ACS) recommends a diet based on a high consumption of plant foods, including fruits, vegetables, grains, and beans, and a low intake of meat, dairy, and other high-fat foods. The ACS also recommends regular exercise and not smoking.

Here are some examples of colon cancer research:

- A Japanese study showed that eating soybeans and tofu lowered the risk of colon cancer by 40 percent.
- A Chinese study showed that people who rarely ate soy products had three times greater risk of colon cancer than people who ate soy regularly.
- In another soy study, men who ate thirty-nine grams of soy protein each day for one year had fewer colon cancer cells in the process of dividing than men who didn't eat soy.

Prostate Cancer

Soy may also have a protective effect against prostate cancer. Epidemiological studies have shown that Asian men who eat soy have lower incidences of and death rates from prostate cancer than their Western counterparts.

Prostate cancer is the second leading cancer for men in the United States. More than 30,000 men in the United States will die from prostate cancer this year, and another 180,400 will be diagnosed. The death rate for prostate cancer is rising, especially for African-American males. The American Cancer Society estimates that almost 19 percent of American men will develop prostate cancer at some time in their life.

When a cancerous tumor forms in the body, a process called angiogenesis occurs, which means that new blood vessels develop to nourish the tumor. Researchers have discovered that the soy isoflavone genistein prevents this process. Without its blood supply, the tumor cannot receive nutrition or oxygen that it needs to grow, nor can it metastasize (send cancerous cells through the bloodstream to other parts of the body).

Additionally, researchers theorize that because prostate cancer can be a hormone-dependent cancer, the isoflavones in soy foods might play a role in interfering with the disease process, thereby lowering risk.

Following are some examples of research results:

- A long-term Hawaiian study showed that eight thousand men of Japanese descent who ate tofu daily were only one-third as likely to develop prostate cancer as men who ate tofu once a week.

- One study showed that the isoflavone genistein slowed the growth of human prostate tumors that had been grafted onto rats.
- Researchers have shown in test tube studies and in some animal studies that isoflavones slow the growth of prostate cells.
- An animal study showed that the incidence of cancer was reduced in rats fed a diet high in isoflavones before exposure to cancer. (And there was a 27 percent increase in the disease-free period.)
- A study showed that genistein inhibited the growth of prostate cancer and reduced metastases.

Breast Cancer

While a number of studies, including many epidemiological studies, have shown that soy may reduce the risk of breast cancer, soy's role in fighting breast cancer has not been fully determined.

Breast cancer is one of the most common types of cancer

among American women. It's estimated that this year more than 182,000 women will be stricken with the disease, and 41,200 people (40,800 women and 400 men) will die from it.

Fifty to 60 percent of breast cancers are hormone-dependent. High levels of the hormone estrogen in the body increase the risk for breast cancer. One theory in breast cancer research is that soy isoflavones can behave as antiestrogens in the body. In other words, the isoflavones can block the actions of the body's estrogen, thereby reducing the risk of breast cancer.

Research has shown that consuming soy foods may provide protective effects against cancer.

- One epidemiological study showed that in premenopausal women, high intakes of animal protein were associated with increased cancer risk and high intakes of soy foods were associated with decreased risk.
- A long-term epidemiological study showed that in pre-menopausal women who regularly consumed miso soup there was a lower breast cancer occurrence.

Some studies in which isoflavones were consumed in the absence of soy protein have yielded different results. In one animal study, the isoflavone genistein did not protect mice from breast cancer, and in others, genistein increased cancer in the animals tested. A British study found that in premenopausal women who consumed forty-five milligrams of isoflavones every day for two weeks, epithelial breast cells were stimulated to proliferate. A similar U.S. study showed proliferation in women drinking soy beverages containing thirty-eight milligrams of isoflavones. These results lead researchers to believe that soy isoflavones are most beneficial to the body when consumed with soy protein. These findings also demonstrate the complicated nature of soy research in relation to chronic diseases and show that researchers still have more work to do in determining which substances in soy provide health benefits.

A University of Illinois study has raised questions about how and when soy may provide protective effects against breast cancer. Researchers found that in mice that were fed isoflavones before they were exposed to cancer, the isoflavones suppressed the cancer. In mice that were fed isoflavones after exposure to cancer, isoflavones seemed to stimulate tumor growth.

Based on this study, researchers have theorized that for women, when soy is consumed might make a difference in its potential protective effects. For example, young women who have grown up eating soy foods before puberty may benefit from protective effects, but postmenopausal women who consume soy may increase their risk of developing certain types of tumors. The difference between the two situations is the amount of estrogen in the body during the various life stages. For this reason, researchers suggest that women who have or have had hormone-dependent breast cancer or have a mother, sister, or aunt who has had hormone-dependent breast cancer avoid using soy supplements, which can contain high concentrations of isoflavones.

Menopause

Soy's role in treating mild to moderate menopausal symptoms looks promising. Epidemiological research has shown that Japanese women, whose typical diet includes soy protein, report fewer and less severe menopausal symptoms than their Western counterparts. In fact, there is no word in the Japanese language for "hot flashes."

Millions of women suffer from the side effects of menopause: hot flashes, night sweats, mood swings, and disrupted sleep. In addition to these uncomfortable symptoms, the loss of estrogen that occurs with menopause can have more serious results. Estrogen plays an important role in keeping bones healthy and it has a protective effect on the heart. The drop in estrogen during menopause leaves women susceptible to osteoporosis, a gradual decay of the bones. Estrogen loss also has an effect on heart health. The rate of heart disease rises in menopausal women, becoming equal to the rate of men.

Estrogen replacement therapy (ERT) and hormone replacement therapy (HRT) are common treatments for reducing menopausal symptoms and the risk of osteoporosis, although many women choose or are advised not to use them. The primary reasons women don't take ERT or HRT is that they think they don't need these treatments or they fear that the treatments will increase their risk of developing breast or endometrial cancer.

Although soy has not been determined to be a complete replacement for hormone replacement therapy, it has been shown to reduce the occurrence and severity of hot flashes.

Because the isoflavones in soy function as weak estrogens, researchers believe that these plant estrogens may take on the role of estrogen when the natural loss of this hormone occurs.

In other words, the plant estrogen stands in and functions like estrogen, thereby lowering the risk of problems like heart disease and bone loss that are associated with low estrogen levels.

Here are a few examples of menopause studies:

- In one study, consuming soy protein reduced the severity of hot flashes, caused minor improvements in the severity of night sweats, reduced cholesterol, and lowered diastolic blood pressure.
- A study revealed that women who consumed soy protein for twelve weeks showed a 45 percent reduction in hot flashes compared with 30 percent who were given a placebo.
- In another study, soy consumption reduced the severity of hot flashes (but was not as effective as hormone replacement therapy) but did not have an effect on vaginal dryness.
- In several studies, women were given soy protein drinks. One study showed that if the beverage was consumed twice a day, the severity of hot flashes was reduced. Another study showed that women drinking soy beverages

experienced fewer hot flashes. In studies using soy flour baked into bars, muffins, or bread, the results women reported were no better than with the placebo.

As with all the health topics mentioned here, more research is needed to determine how soy affects health and fights disease. For women who experience side effects from ERT or HRT or believe ERT and HRT to be unnecessary or unsafe, soy provides some relief of menopausal symptoms without side effects.

Osteoporosis

Studies suggest that soy protein with naturally occurring isoflavones has positive effects on bone mineral density.

Osteoporosis is a bone disease characterized by the deterioration of bone tissue that eventually leaves bones fragile and susceptible to fractures. More than 10 million Americans have osteoporosis; 80 percent of them are women. Another 18 million people are at risk for osteoporosis.

In healthy bones a balance is maintained; bone cells called

osteoblasts create bone tissue, and other cells called osteoclasts break down, or resorb, bone tissue. The drop in estrogen levels that occurs with menopause can disrupt this dynamic. For some reason, new bone cells stop being created, but osteoclasts continue to resorb bone, resulting in bone loss that can leave bones weak and brittle.

Studies have focused on determining whether reducing animal protein and increasing plant protein affects bone health. High intakes of animal protein are associated with calcium loss and bone resorption. Researchers have discovered that soy protein does not cause calcium loss or bone resorption to occur, making soy a beneficial food for bone health.

Here are two samples of bone studies:

- In a University of Illinois study, postmenopausal women consumed soy protein with ninety milligrams of isoflavones every day for six months. After six months, the women had higher bone mineral density in their lumbar spines; other bones showed no difference. (Minerals are more quickly absorbed into the spine.)
- In vitro and animal studies have shown that genistein stopped bone loss.

OTHER HEALTH CONCERNS

Diabetes

As early as 1900, soy was suggested as a good food for diabetics by two doctors who published their recommendations in the *American Journal of Medical Science.* Several years later, Dr. John Kellogg, who eventually built a breakfast cereal empire around cornflakes, wrote about the beneficial effects of eating soy foods for diabetics. For the 10.3 million Americans who have diabetes (and another 5.4 million who have it and have not yet been diagnosed), soy, as part of a low-fat diet, can help increase fiber intake, regulate blood sugar, lower blood pressure, and reduce the risk of heart disease by lowering high cholesterol.

Diabetes is a disease that disrupts the normal functioning and utilization of insulin in the body. Insulin is necessary to convert sugar and starch into the energy your body needs to function every day. When insulin doesn't function normally, sugar builds up in the bloodstream, causing fatigue, blood circulation problems, nerve damage in the feet, and even blindness in severe cases. Regulating this process is essential for diabetics to remain healthy.

Health Benefits of Soy

Diet and weight control play a key role in treating diabetes. One way diabetics maintain a healthy blood sugar level is to pay attention to the glycemic index of foods. In the glycemic index, foods are rated based on how they affect blood sugar levels. Soy is low on the index, which means that it is beneficial in maintaining stable blood sugar levels. Soy is also believed to help slow down the absorption of sugars.

Diabetics often have high blood pressure and increased risk of heart attack (diabetics are four times more likely than the general population to develop heart disease), stroke, and kidney disease.

Research has focused on looking at soy's role in reducing cholesterol (to provide protective heart-health benefits) and helping maintain stable blood sugar.

Here are two study findings:

- Diabetic subjects who consumed twenty-five grams of soy fiber a day had a reduced insulin response to an oral glucose challenge and had a reduced total plasma cholesterol level.
- Soy may prevent kidney damage by lowering blood cholesterol levels.

Allergies

According to the following research findings compiled by the United Soybean Board, soy might be an answer for many people with food allergies, although, like many subjects, not all researchers agree.

The incidence of food allergies is fairly low in the U.S. population (only 1 to 2 percent of adults and 5 to 8 percent of children have food allergies), but these allergies should be taken very seriously because they can cause dangerous reactions in some people. Some of the most common foods to which people are allergic include cow's milk, eggs, peanuts, wheat, and shellfish. For people with food allergies, soy foods can provide a tasty alternative. Soy milk can stand in for cow's milk, scrambled tofu for eggs, and soy nuts for peanuts.

For babies allergic to cow's milk, soy milk can provide the necessary nutrients babies need to grow and develop. Used in infant formulas since the 1920s, processed soy has improved greatly over the past seventy years. Today's formulas contain protein equal in quality and digestibility to cow's milk. Research has also demonstrated that babies fed soy formula experience normal growth rates.

Health Benefits of Soy

While soy is a common ingredient in many formulas, researchers do not always agree on how to treat babies with cow's-milk allergies. Based on the belief that infants with cow's-milk allergy might suffer intestinal damage that would also make them likely to develop an allergy to soy milk, the American Academy of Pediatrics recommends that allergy-prone babies who are formula fed should not be switched to soy formula after demonstrating an allergy to cow's milk. Some researchers disagree with this recommendation and believe that soy milk can be used after a cow's-milk allergy has been discovered.

Although allergies to animal proteins are more common, some people are allergic to soy. Because soy foods are processed in a variety of ways, some soy foods are less allergenic than others. In general, foods that have been heated or fermented, like tofu, tempeh, and miso, are less allergenic than raw soy foods like soybeans and soy sprouts. With any food allergy, it is important to read food labels carefully to determine whether the products you buy contain substances to which you might be allergic.

SOY AND BRAIN HEALTH

The small amount of research that has been done on soy and brain health indicates that soy may have beneficial effects in the brain. Like the heart and bones, the brain requires estrogen to maintain normal health and function and can be affected by the natural reduction of estrogen women experience during menopause. A small percentage of women, due to a variety of environmental, hereditary, or other factors that may include estrogen reduction during menopause, may be at risk of developing cognitive dysfunction, and even Alzheimer's, later in life.

As you read earlier in this chapter, soy isoflavones sometimes act like estrogen in the body and sometimes they act like antiestrogens. Research has looked at the possibility that soy isoflavones can "stand in" for estrogen, positively affecting cognitive function.

Study findings include:

- Female rats whose ovaries were removed (thereby reducing estrogen levels in their bodies) gradually became cognitively impaired. Female rats that were fed soy isoflavones after their ovaries were removed did not lose their cognitive abilities. The effects were the same if they were given estrogen in their diets.

- In studies using monkeys, an animal model closer to humans than either rats or mice, researchers found that eating soy prevented certain chemical changes in brain proteins that may be involved in the development of Alzheimer's disease.

ISOFLAVONES IN SOY FOODS

How do you know which soy foods contain isoflavones and how much of these foods to eat to gain health benefits?

Sometimes it's difficult to find the isoflavone content of foods because many food manufacturers don't list this information on their food labels. With soy research becoming more publicized, manufacturers will probably begin to include this information. What researchers aren't clear on yet is whether soy foods are more potent when soy protein and soy isoflavones are eaten together. However, many researchers agree that the best source of the potential disease-fighting benefits come from whole soy foods with naturally occurring isoflavones. Highly processed soy foods, like powdered protein drink mixes, may contain the highest protein and isoflavone contents, but the processing of these products removes or weakens their potency.

Is soy safe to eat?

Eating soy is healthy and safe. There has been no indication that eating soy foods causes cancer or affects fertility. Researchers do caution against using soy supplements (isoflavone capsules) because these substances are not regulated by the FDA, nor have researchers yet determined a maximum isoflavone intake. As mentioned above, researchers recommend eating whole soy foods to gain the benefits of soy protein with naturally occurring isoflavones. In other words, because it's not yet clear if there is any risk of toxicity at high levels, you might want to stick to eating soy foods to get your isoflavones. It could be possible for someone to unwittingly take too many pills, but it's unlikely that a person would eat too much soy. As you can see in the chart on page 11 and in the recipes in chapter 5, a serving size of soy is often just one-half to one cup.

Health Benefits of Soy

How much isoflavones do I need to eat to gain health benefits?

Asian women (that is, living in Asian countries and consuming the typical Asian diet), who experience lower rates of menopause symptoms, heart disease, and some cancers, consume between twenty and eighty milligrams of isoflavones a day, compared with less than five milligrams consumed daily by U.S. women.

While there are no government recommendations or regulations for soy isoflavones, based on two research studies, one in China and one in Japan, some of the top U.S. soy researchers recommend sixty milligrams a day. The FDA's recommendation of twenty-five grams of soy protein a day for cholesterol-lowering benefits does not include an isoflavone value. It's difficult to know how much isoflavones are in that twenty-five grams. Some soy foods contain more isoflavones than others. For example, soybeans, tempeh, and tofu all contain high amounts of isoflavones and soy protein.

The chart on the next page lists many soy foods and their isoflavone content. The isoflavone contents are based on mean values and have been rounded to the nearest whole number. Please note that isoflavone content in soy foods can vary greatly from brand to brand depending on how the products are processed by food manufacturers. Also, this chart is based on milligrams of isoflavones per 100 grams of food. It's difficult to convert grams to an exact serving size like one-half or one cup. You can approximate measurements in grams as follows: 250 grams is roughly equal to one cup.

ISOFLAVONE CONTENT OF SOY FOODS	
Soy food	**Isoflavones in mg per 100 g of food**
Soybean oil	0
Soybean butter	1
Soy cheese, cheddar	7
Soy cheese, mozzarella	8
Soy cheese, Parmesan	6
Soy hot dog, unprepared	15
Soy veggie patty, cooked (Green Giant brand)	8
Soy sprouts	41
Soybeans, green, immature, cooked w/o salt	14
Soybeans, green, mature, cooked w/o salt	55
Soybeans, mature, roasted	128

Health Benefits of Soy

Soy food	Isoflavones in mg per 100 g of food
Soy milk	10
Soy sauce made from soy and wheat (shoyu)	2
Soy sauce made from hydrolyzed vegetable protein	0
Soy breakfast sausage links (Morningstar Farms brand), cooked	4
Tempeh, cooked	53
Tofu, silken, firm (Mori-Nu brand)	28
Tofu, silken, soft (Vitasoy brand)	29
Miso	43
Tofu yogurt	16
Soy flour (full-fat, roasted)	199
Soy protein isolate	97
Natto	59
Yuba, cooked	51

(Source: 1999 USDA Iowa State University Database on Isoflavone Content of Food)

Using this chart and the chart on page 11, you'll see that it's not difficult to get your daily soy protein and soy isoflavone values. If you eat a salad topped with soy nuts for lunch and a tofu stir-fry for dinner, you'll easily meet the recommended twenty-five grams of protein and sixty milligrams of isoflavones.

Who benefits from eating soy?

With the exception of people who have soy allergies, both children and adults can benefit from eating soy. Soy is a nutritious, low-fat, cholesterol-free food that provides fiber and high-quality protein. For millions of Americans trying to decrease their fat and cholesterol intake and increase their consumption of plant-based foods, soy provides a healthy, tasty alternative to higher-fat meat and dairy products.

In addition to soy's role as a low-fat, high-protein food source, soy contains disease-fighting substances that appear to be useful in preventing or slowing down disease processes. As you read in this chapter, some people that might benefit from eating soy as part of a low-fat diet include:

- People with high cholesterol
- People at risk of colorectal cancer
- Men at risk of prostate cancer
- Women at risk of breast cancer
- Women experiencing menopausal symptoms and who are at risk of developing osteoporosis

- Menopausal women who choose not to take hormone replacement therapy

It is important to clarify that researchers are not recommending that people eat only soy. One food alone is not a cure-all, nor does it make for a healthy diet. To gain the essential nutrients required, you need to eat a variety of foods. In fact, it may be the synthesis of several foods in combination that provides protective effects.

To maintain a healthy lifestyle and help prevent disease, researchers recommend a balanced approach that includes exercising regularly, not smoking, and eating a nutritious low-fat diet that includes many different foods, especially fruits and vegetables. As with any changes in your diet or exercise routine, it's always important to discuss your plans with your doctor.

4 Soy Foods

Adding soy to your diet is easy. Whether it's roasted vegetable veggie burgers, creamy chocolate soy milk, or spicy breakfast sausages you hunger for, there are so many different types of soy foods that you shouldn't have any trouble finding foods that you like.

Many soy products, like soy milk, veggie burgers, tofu, miso, and soy meat alternatives, are widely available at supermarkets across the country. Other soy products can be found at natural food stores, Asian markets, and mail order companies.

More than twenty soy foods, in seven categories, are listed in this chapter—common soy foods that you've probably heard of and eaten before; traditional soy foods like tofu, tempeh, and miso; whole-bean soy foods; soy dairy products; soy flour and soy grits; soy in processed foods; and other soy foods. Many of the foods could be listed under more than one category; I've designated categories to make it easier for readers to find information about specific foods.

I've also listed brand names for several of the products. These suggestions are not endorsements but merely guides to help you familiarize yourself with products so that you know what to look for in the store. As with all food products you buy, read labels carefully. Soy is a nutritious low-fat food, but products that are highly processed may contain high amounts of fat, sugar, or salt. In other words, just because a product contains soy doesn't mean it's healthy. To gain health benefits, look for soy foods with the least amount of processing.

COMMON SOY FOODS

Soy milk, soy oil, soy sauce, and soy meat alternatives like deli meats and hot dogs are some of the most common and widely available soy foods.

Soy Milk

Creamy and delicious, soy milk is a tasty low-fat, lactose-free alternative to cow's milk and one of the easiest soy foods to incorporate into your diet. In recent years soy milk has become one of the most popular soy products. Extracted from pressed soybeans, soy milk is high in protein and B vitamins, rich in calcium, and like many brands of cow's milk, it is fortified with vitamins A and D (some manufacturers also add vitamin B_{12}). Depending on the manufacturer, soy milk can range in color from white to light brown.

Widely available at supermarkets and natural food stores, soy milk can be found in the milk section and in the cereal or baking aisles (many brands are sold in special shelf-stable containers that do not require refrigeration). Some brands, like Edensoy, package soy milk in individual juice-box size (eight ounces). Unopened, soy milk in shelf-stable packaging can be kept in the cupboard for five or six months. Once opened, soy milk must be stored in the refrigerator, where it will stay fresh for up to a week.

You can drink soy milk as you would cow's milk. It has a creamy texture and comes in flavors like vanilla, chocolate, strawberry, and mocha. You can also add it to coffee, tea, and smoothies, or pour it over your breakfast cereal. Like cow's milk, soy milk is available in nonfat, low-fat, and 2 percent fat varieties, although nonfat soy milk can taste pretty watery. You're better off sticking with the 2 percent or regular soy milk, which still contains only one-half gram of saturated fat per serving. While soy is a common ingredient in infant formula, soy milk itself should not be used as infant formula.

Some brands to look for include Vitasoy, Westbrae, Silk (in the refrigerated section), Pacific Foods, Edensoy, Trader Joe's Soy Um.

COOKING WITH SOY MILK

Soy milk can be used in recipes to replace cow's milk. Sauces, dressings, and baked goods can all be made with soy milk. (See page 143 for Poppy Seed Dressing and page 118 for Cinnamon Soy Pancakes).

Soy milk powder mixed with water can also be used as an egg replacer.

Soybean Oil

Seventy-five percent of the vegetable oil consumed in the United States is soybean oil, which is extracted from soybeans. Light tasting and virtually odorless, soybean oil is low in saturated fat, high in polyunsaturated fat, and cholesterol-free. It also contains a blend of omega-3 and omega-6 fatty acids, similar to the fatty acids found in fish, which are believed to be beneficial to heart health.

You'll find soybean oil shelved with other oils. You may already be using soy oil and not know it. Read the labels of your favorite vegetable oils to see if they are 100 percent soy oil. Soy oil is also used by food manufacturers to make margarine, mayonnaise, salad dressings, and coffee creamers. Unopened soy oil can be stored in the cupboard. Once opened, it should be stored in the refrigerator.

COOKING WITH SOYBEAN OIL

Soy oil is ideal for cooking because its neutral taste allows the flavors of foods cooked in it to come through. Its high smoking point (440°F) makes it a great oil to use when frying at high temperatures.

Soy Sauce

Traditional soy sauce, called shoyu, is made by mixing soybeans with a grain, like wheat, and a mold culture and fermenting the mixture for at least a year. Tamari sauce, a by-product of miso, is made from fermented soybeans without the added grain. Teriyaki sauce has a thicker consistency than soy sauce and contains ingredients like sugar and vinegar. The soy sauce that most Americans buy at the store is generally not fermented and may contain chemicals, coloring, and other additives.

Soy sauce is typically used as a garnish to top Asian dishes, in salad dressings, and in marinades. All soy sauces are high in sodium, so use them sparingly. You'll find soy sauces in the Asian-foods section of the grocery store. Once opened, soy sauce should be stored in the refrigerator.

COOKING WITH SOY SAUCE

Use soy sauces to flavor vegetable and meat dishes as well as soups, stir-fries, and stews.

> Soybean oil is the most frequently consumed vegetable oil in the United States and the number one vegetable oil consumed in the world.

Soy Meat Alternatives

For people who are trying to lower their saturated fat intake but don't want to give up that meaty taste, soy meat alternatives are the perfect choice. They are similar in appearance, smell, taste, and texture to their animal-protein counterparts, without the cholesterol and saturated fat. Choose among soy-based hamburgers, ground round, hot dogs, spicy Italian sausages, breakfast links and patties, chicken and turkey breasts, chicken nuggets, deli meat slices (ham, turkey, beef, bologna), Canadian bacon, pepperoni, salmon, tuna, and even corn dogs! Eat soy meats as you would other meats: in sandwiches and casseroles, on top of pizza, or with potatoes, rice, or pasta.

Soy meat alternatives are made from a variety of soy foods, including soybeans, tofu, textured soy protein, and other ingredients. In general, these products contain less saturated fat and cholesterol than beef or other meats, although nutritional values differ among brands. Read the labels carefully; some soy "meats" can be very high in fat and sodium and may not contain isoflavones. Look for soy meat alternatives in the refrigerated and frozen meat sections. Store soy meat in the refrigerator or freezer, according to instructions on the package label.

The quality and taste of soy meat alternatives vary among products; try a few different brands to find the products you like best. Some brands to look for include Lightlife Italian Links, Yves Veggie Ground Round, Boca Burgers, Morningstar Farms, and Lightlife Gimme Lean.

COOKING WITH SOY MEATS

Add soy meats to recipes as you would other meats. Follow instructions that come with the product. Some soy meats will need to be browned or heated before use; others can be used right from the package.

Substitute soy meats for all or part of the meat in your favorite dishes. For example, instead of eating scrambled eggs with sausages or bacon, try tofu scramble with soy breakfast patties or links. You can use veggie ground round instead of ground beef when making chili or topping a pizza.

When replacing part of the meat in a recipe with a soy meat alternative, using spices, garlic, or other seasonings can unify the taste of the two meats.

TRADITIONAL SOY FOODS

Tofu, tempeh, and miso, all traditional staples in Asian countries, may sound exotic, but they're actually very versatile and simple foods to prepare. You should be able to find these foods at your local supermarket.

Tofu

Tofu, also called soybean curd, is made from curdled soy milk (similar to the way cheese is made from curdled cow's milk). The curds are pressed into rectangular white blocks, or cakes. Tofu comes in three main varieties, firm, soft, and silken. Firm tofu has a rubbery texture and is spongy on the inside. Soft tofu looks more like thick custard, and silken tofu is smooth and creamy like a thick yogurt.

A great source of protein, iron, and calcium, tofu is also one of the most versatile soy foods. You'll find tofu in the refrigerated-foods section. Some brands of tofu are packaged in shelf-stable packaging and therefore don't require refrigeration until opened.

Tofu comes in a variety of styles, including plain, marinated, hickory smoked, seasoned, garlic-and-onion flavored, and baked. Some brands to look for include Nasoya, Mori-Nu, White Wave, Smoke & Fire, and Azumaya.

Store tofu in the refrigerator. Once you've opened the package, store tofu in a loosely sealed container of water for up to a week, changing the water every day. If the tofu smells bad, throw it out. Unused tofu can also be frozen for up to five months. Once frozen, it will become chewier and change to a light brown color.

Cooking with Tofu

Cooking with tofu is simple. Alone, it has a bland, neutral taste, but as you cook it, tofu absorbs the flavors of the sauce, vegetables, and other ingredients in the recipe. You can mash it and scramble it with herbs for breakfast, cut it into small cubes and add it to miso soup for lunch, or sauté rectangles of tofu with broccoli in black bean sauce for dinner (see recipe on page 156). Tofu can be marinated, baked, fried, grilled, and steamed. Blend silken tofu into smoothies or puree it into sauces. If you're not convinced that tofu can be delicious, try the Chocolate Raspberry Truffle Pie recipe on page 102.

Here are a few other cooking tips for tofu:

- Mix it with ground beef to replace some of the meat in lasagna or casseroles.
- Use firm tofu when you want the tofu to hold its shape. Firm tofu works best in soups, casseroles, and stir-fries and for grilling.
- Soft tofu is good for soups and in recipes that include blended tofu.
- Silken tofu, which is creamier and looks like firm yogurt, is great for smoothies, dips and sauces, and desserts. Use it whenever you want to make something creamy. Pureed silken tofu can be used as a substitute for part of the sour cream, cream cheese, ricotta cheese, or mayonnaise in recipes.

Tempeh (TEM-pay)

Tempeh is a soybean loaf or cake made from whole soybeans. Traditionally, tempeh was made by mixing soybeans with a grain (rice or millet), wrapping the mixture in banana leaves, and fermenting it for a few days. In Indonesia, where tempeh is a staple food, it is eaten as a snack food and with rice. Tempeh usually comes packaged in a rectangular block, similar to tofu.

High in protein and vitamin B_{12} and rich in calcium, tempeh has a nutty flavor, and like tofu, it absorbs the flavors of the foods with which it is cooked. Don't be put off by its appearance; the thin, flaky outer covering of this whole-bean cake is just a by-product of the fermentation process. It is perfectly safe to eat.

Tempeh can be found with the frozen foods or in the refrigerated section, with tofu and miso. Tempeh comes in many different styles, like vegetable, five-grain, and wild rice. You can also find marinated tempeh, smoked tempeh, and grilled tempeh. Its chewy texture makes tempeh an ideal substitute for meat in stir-fries and other dishes, and it goes well with rice. Some brands to look for include Smoke & Fire, Lightlife, Turtle Island Foods, and White Wave.

Store tempeh in the refrigerator. Once opened, it will stay fresh for about ten days.

COOKING WITH TEMPEH

Tempeh needs to be cooked before it is eaten. Like meat, it can be marinated, cut into chunks, grilled, and sautéed. Tempeh can also be steamed. Use the flavored tempeh chunks in wraps, vegetable dishes, and burritos, and add them to sauces and stews (see page 158 for Curried Red Lentil Stew with Tempeh). If you are adding tempeh to a stew that will be simmering, you do not need to precook it.

Miso

A staple in Japanese cooking, miso is a salty paste made from soybeans that are mixed with a grain—usually rice or barley—salt, and koji (a mold culture that aids in the fermentation process) and aged in cedar vats for up to three years. Miso has a texture like peanut butter and comes in a range of colors and flavors, from light to dark, subtle to strong.

A high-sodium, high-protein food, miso is 12 to 21 percent

protein, which is similar to the protein content of chicken (20 percent). This highly concentrated paste is used (in small amounts) to flavor soups, sauces, and vegetable dishes.

Miso is usually sold in plastic containers similar to yogurt containers and can be found in the refrigerated section, often in the same place as tofu. Miso comes in pasteurized or unpasteurized varieties. Store miso in a sealed container in the refrigerator.

COOKING WITH MISO

Light misos like white or yellow miso have a subtle, almost sweet taste and are generally milder and less salty than darker misos, like red miso, which are saltier and have a heartier, earthy flavor.

Hatcho (hot-cho) miso is the most revered miso in Japan, with its own unique traditions. This dark brown miso is made using a special type of mold and aged longer than other misos.

Here are a few additional cooking tips for miso:

- Before adding miso to a soup or sauce, dilute it in a little bit of water or broth from the soup to help it dissolve.

- Add miso to soup near the end of the cooking time and do not boil the soup, because boiling can destroy the properties of the miso and turn the soup bitter.
- Miso can be very salty; you may want to taste your soup before you add ingredients like salt or soy sauce.
- Miso paste can be substituted for anchovy paste.

WHOLE SOYBEANS

The possibilities for soybeans seem endless. They can be cooked, boiled, roasted, ground, and sprouted.

Soybeans

Soybeans are pea-sized legumes that grow in pods on the soybean plant and come in three main varieties: yellow, brown, and black. They can be used in salads and chilis and even served alone as a tasty snack. A great source of calcium, soybeans also have a higher protein content than other beans.

There is a controversy about genetically modified foods,

crops that have been bred to withstand threats from bugs or other plants that might destroy a crop. Fifty to 60 percent of soybeans are genetically modified, although nongenetically modified soybeans are available.

Organic soybeans are grown without the use of chemical pesticides. You can find organic soybeans at natural food stores. Read package labels, or ask a salesperson at your grocery store, to find out what types of soybeans you are buying. Generally, companies that use nongenetically modified or organic soybeans will label their packages accordingly.

Whole soybeans are available at health food stores and co-ops as well as at some supermarkets. Some of the whole-bean products available are dry soybeans sold in bulk, canned soybeans (yellow and black), and roasted soybeans (called soy nuts). Fermented black soybeans, can also be found in the Asian-foods section of your supermarket. Some brands to look for include Edensoy canned black soybeans, Hain canned soybeans, Sun Luck and Lee Kum Kee bean sauces.

Cooked soybeans can be used as you would use other beans. Add them to soups, stews, chili, burritos, and casseroles. Black bean sauce can be used in a stir-fry with vegetables, tofu, and shrimp (see recipe on page 156). Canned soybeans can be stored in the cupboard. Dried beans should be stored in an air-tight container. Black bean sauce, once opened, must be stored in the refrigerator.

COOKING WITH SOYBEANS

- Using canned soybeans in recipes is much quicker and easier than soaking and cooking dried beans. One fifteen-ounce can of soybeans (yellow or black) is the equivalent of one and one-half cups of cooked soybeans.
- Rinsing canned soybeans in water before use will reduce their sodium content by 40 percent.
- Dry soybeans have to be soaked and cooked before use. If you do want to use dry soybeans, first pick out the stones and broken beans. Then rinse the beans with water and soak them (four cups of water per cup of beans) overnight. Drain the water and add fresh cooking water (the same amount you used for soaking), and bring it to a boil. Once the water boils, skim off the foam that forms on the surface, reduce the heat, and simmer the beans for about three hours (one and one-half hours for black soybeans), adding more water if necessary. Stop cooking the beans

when they are tender. You can also cook beans in a pressure cooker in about thirty minutes.

Edamame (eh-dah-mah-meh)

Edamame are soybeans that have been harvested just before reaching full maturity. These large green beans have a sweet flavor and are a favorite snack food in Japan.

Boiled or steamed, edamame can be added to stir-fries or sprinkled on salads (see Protein-Power Dinner Salad on page 145). Lightly salted edamame beans make a fresh, healthy, high-protein snack. Pop the beans into your mouth right from the pod. (Edamame beans should be boiled in salty water for about five minutes before serving. Do not eat the pods; they are hard to digest.) Edamame are usually found in the freezer section in shelled and unshelled varieties, and sometimes you can buy them precooked. Store uncooked edamame in the freezer.

Soy Nuts

Soy nuts, also called roasted soybeans, are soybeans that have been roasted in oil or dry roasted. They are light and crispy—

perfect as a topping for salads, yogurt, and ice cream or as a snack food (see page 106 for Fun Fruity Parfaits). Just one one-half-cup serving of soy nuts provides the twenty-five grams of soy protein recommended by the FDA for cholesterol-lowering effects.

Soy nuts are higher in protein than peanuts and a good source of isoflavones. The roasting process adds fat, so soy nuts are not low in fat like most soy foods. The nutritional value of soy nuts may vary from brand to brand. Soy nuts can be found in the snacks aisle with the pretzels and chips.

Soy Nut Butter

Soy nut butter is made from ground roasted soybeans. It has the same texture and consistency as peanut butter, with a rich, nutty taste. Soy nut butter is high in protein, and while not a low-fat food, it has one-third less fat than peanut butter.

Soy nut butter comes in jars just like peanut butter and can be found in the same section as peanut butter and other nut butters. Eat soy nut butter the same way you eat peanut butter: on crackers or bread and in cooking. See page 110 for Nut

Butter Balls, a sweet, crunchy snack. Store soy nut butter in the cupboard. Once opened, it should be refrigerated.

Cooking with Soy Nut Butter

Soy nut butter can be used in recipes to make sauces, cookies, and desserts (see Spicy Soba Noodles with Soy Nuts on page 137).

Soy Sprouts

Just like other beans and seeds, soybeans can be sprouted. It takes about a week for the beans to sprout. Soy sprouts are high in protein and vitamin C and can be used like mung bean sprouts or alfalfa sprouts: put them in sandwiches and salads. You'll find soy sprouts in the produce section with other sprouts.

Cooking Sprouts

Soy sprouts should be cooked (with other food) quickly on low heat to prevent them from wilting. Add them to soups, stews, or stir-fries during the final minute of cooking.

TOP TEN AVAILABLE SOY FOODS

Soy sauce
Soybean oil
Tofu
Miso
Soy milk
Soy meat alternatives
Soy cheese, yogurt, ice cream
Roasted soy nuts
Soy protein powder
Soy nutrition bars

SOY DAIRY

Who doesn't love cheese sprinkled on almost any dish or enjoy an ice-cream cone on a hot day? Dairy products are some of the most enjoyable foods to eat, but unfortunately they're also loaded with saturated fat and cholesterol. For people who want to enjoy dairy without the guilt and for people with lactose intolerance, soy dairy products, which look and taste like ice cream, yogurt, and cheese made from cow's milk, are great alternatives. Other soy products available include soy cream cheese, soy sour cream, and soy coffee creamer (with flavors like amaretto and French vanilla).

Soy Ice Cream

Soy ice cream tastes rich and creamy, just like cow's-milk ice cream. It's delicious on its own, topped with fruit and soy nuts, or blended into a shake. Soy ice cream can be lower in fat than ice cream, but isn't always. Read the labels to find the brands that work best for you. Soy ice cream can be found in the frozen foods section of the grocery store, just like regular ice cream. Store soy ice cream, and other frozen soy treats in the freezer. Some products to look for include Tofutti brand ice cream and ice-cream sandwiches, Soy Delicious ice cream, and Dairylike frozen dessert.

Soy Yogurt

Soy yogurt is made from soy milk, just like yogurt is made from cow's milk. Creamy in texture and available in many different flavors, soy yogurt is high in protein (twelve grams per cup) and low in fat. For a high-power breakfast, add soy yogurt, topped with fruit and soy nuts, to your morning menu. Soy yogurt can also be used to replace sour cream or cream cheese, both high in fat; as a topping or dip; and in sauces, dressings, and baked goods. Like cow's-milk yogurt, soy yogurt should be stored in the refrigerator. Once opened, it stays fresh for five to seven days.

Soy Cheese

Like soy yogurt, soy cheese is made from soy milk. It resembles cheese in appearance, but has a milder taste. Soy cheese comes in many varieties and flavors, including cheddar, hickory smoked, mozzarella, Parmesan, provolone, and Swiss. Cholesterol-free and lower in fat than cow's-milk cheese, soy cheese is available in regular and low-fat styles. Vegans should be aware that most soy cheeses contain a milk protein called casein. Casein-free vegan soy cheese is also available.

Soy Foods

Soy cheeses can be found in the dairy section with other cheeses, or in special natural foods sections. Store soy cheese in the refrigerator. Eat soy cheese the same way you would eat cow's-milk cheese: Slice it and serve on crackers or in sandwiches, grate it and sprinkle on pasta, and mix it into lasagnas and casseroles. Soy cream cheese can be used as a substitute for regular cream cheese. Some brands to look for include Soya Kass, TofuRella (both were used in the recipes in chapter 5), and Galaxy Foods Veggie Slices and Veggie Cream Cheese.

COOKING WITH SOY CHEESE

Soy cheese can be used in combination with, or to replace, cow's-milk cheese. Use soy mozzarella on pizzas, soy Parmesan on pasta dishes, and soy cheddar in burritos and sandwiches. Some soy cheese, such as cream cheese, may separate when cooked, so read labels and follow instructions carefully. Soy cheese used as a topping on baked foods, like pizza or lasagna, should be added near the end of the baking period because cooking it for too long changes its consistency. Overcooked soy cheese can turn into a hard lump that looks like plastic. Soya Kass and TofuRella brand cheeses were used in the recipes in this book (Spinach Lasagna, page 151; Erika's Zucchini and Garlic Pizza, page 149).

Sales of soy milk have grown more than 700 percent in the past decade, with sales reaching $140 million in 1995.

SOY FLOUR AND SOY GRITS

Soy flour can be used to replace a portion of the flour in baked goods. Soy grits, much less common and hard to find, can also be used in baking and cooking. Unless you're really serious about experimenting with many different soy foods, it's not really worth tracking down or using soy grits in cooking.

Soy Flour

Soy flour, made from ground roasted soybeans, can be used in baking to produce moist products that will stay fresh longer than ordinary baked goods. Food manufacturers have long used soy flour, also a source of high-quality protein, for this purpose. There are two main types of soy flour: full-fat, which contains the soybeans' natural oils, and defatted, from which the oils have been removed.

Soy flour can be found in the baking aisle, with other flours. Some brands to look for include Arrowhead Mills (organic) and Trader Joe's. Soy flour is sometimes hard to find, but it can be purchased from mail order companies like Bob's Red Mill Natural Foods (503-654-3215) and Something Better Natural Foods (616-965-1199). Store soy flour in a sealed container, in the refrigerator or freezer.

COOKING WITH SOY FLOUR

You can use soy flour in recipes to boost the soy-protein content. Because soy flour is denser and moister than wheat flour, it cannot be used alone in recipes. Soy flour works well in pancakes, waffles, and muffins, and it can also be used (mixed with water) as an egg replacer (see chart on page 96). Here are some additional cooking tips for soy flour:

- You can replace up to one-fourth of the total amount of flour in a recipe with soy flour for non–yeast-raised baked goods.
- You can replace 15 percent of the flour (wheat or rye) with soy flour in bread recipes. (Because soy is gluten-free, you must use predominantly wheat or rye flour or the bread won't rise.) To calculate 15 percent, place two tablespoons of soy flour into your one-cup measure before adding the rest of the flour.
- When using soy flour in baked goods, you may need to reduce baking time or bake at a lower temperature, because baked foods that contain soy flour brown more quickly.
- Soy flour can settle during packaging. Stir it gently before measuring.

Soy Grits

Soy grits, like soy flour, are made from ground roasted soybeans and are high in protein. Grits are not ground as fine as flour but into tiny flakes or chunks. With so many good soy products available, you may not want to go to the trouble to track down soy grits.

Soy grits can be difficult to find at stores but can be purchased from mail order companies like Bob's Red Mill Natural Foods (503-654-3215) and Something Better Natural Foods (616-965-1199).

Add soy grits to soups or casseroles or mix with ground beef as a meat extender. Grits can also be cooked with grains like rice and with hot cereals.

SOY IN PROCESSED FOODS

Soy contains many nutrients and other substances that food manufacturers use in food processing.

Textured Soy Protein (TSP)

Textured soy protein, also called textured vegetable protein (TVP), is made from soy flour and used as a meat extender or replacer and added to processed foods by the food industry.

TVP can be difficult to find. If your local natural food store does not carry it, you can purchase it from a mail order company like The Mail Order Catalog (800-695-2241) or Something Better Natural Foods (616-965-1199). TVP can be stored in a sealed container in the cupboard for several months. Once rehydrated it should be refrigerated and used within a few days.

Cooking with TVP

TVP can be used to extend the meat in meatballs or meat loaf or replace all or a portion of the meat in dishes like chili and lasagna. It can be added directly to soups and sauces that contain a lot of liquid. For use in other recipes, TVP should be rehydrated. Rehydrate it by pouring seven-eighths of a cup of boiling water over one cup of TVP. Let it sit for a few minutes before mixing it with other ingredients.

Soy Protein Concentrate and Soy Protein Isolate

Both soy protein concentrate and soy protein isolate are made from defatted soy flakes. Soy protein concentrate is about 70 percent protein and still contains fiber. Soy protein isolate, the most refined soy product, is more than 90 percent soy protein, with the fiber removed. You won't find soy protein concentrate in the stores; it is mainly used by food manufacturers as an ingredient in packaged soup and sauce recipes and in other packaged foods. Soy protein isolate is used in baked goods, infant formula, pasta, and soups and is a common ingredient in nutrition bars and in many powdered protein drink mixes that are used in making smoothies, a thick blended drink consisting of fruit, juice, and yogurt.

Hydrolyzed Vegetable Protein (HVP)

Hydrolyzed vegetable protein is a vegetable protein extracted from soybeans or other vegetables. It is not available to consumers but is used by food manufacturers to flavor soups, sauces, canned vegetables, and other food products.

Infant Formula

Soy protein isolate is used in soy-based formulas in place of cow's milk. As a result of processing, soy infant formula may be brown in color and have a strong smell.

Lecithin

Lecithin is a by-product of soybean oil that is used extensively in the food industry as an emulsifier. Emulsifiers are substances that keep the fats in food products (like margarine, ice cream, and chocolate) mixed together with the other ingredients.

OTHER SOY FOODS

The following soy foods are popular in Asian countries but hard to find here.

Natto

Natto is made from fermented soybeans and has a sticky, pasty texture. In Asian countries, natto is eaten as a breakfast and as a dinner food. Natto is used as a topping for rice and added to vegetable dishes and miso soup. You may be able to find natto at Asian markets.

Yuba

Yuba, a popular soy food in China and Japan, is made from the "skin" that forms on the surface of heated soy milk as it cools. Dried sheets of yuba can be deep-fried to make crispy snack chips. Yuba can also be added to soups and stews or used as a wrap. To make wraps, dried yuba sheets are soaked in water to soften them, and then they are wrapped around vegetables or rice. You may be able to find yuba at Asian markets.

Soy Fiber

There are three main types of soy fiber: soy bran, which is made from the hulls (the outer coating) of the soybean; soy isolate fiber (also called structured protein fiber, SPF); and okara, a flaky by-product of soy milk.

Consumers can't buy soy bran or soy isolate fiber in stores. Manufacturers in food processing use these soy products to add fiber to a variety of food products.

Used by the food industry, okara is sometimes an ingredient in veggie burgers, sausages, baked goods, and other soy products. Okara is difficult to find. You may be able to find it at an

Asian food market that makes tofu. Use okara right away; it is very perishable.

SOY FOODS DIRECTORY

For more information about where to find soy products and how to order them through the mail, see the resources section in the back of the book.

5 Cooking with Soy

Soy is one of the most versatile and nutritious foods you can have in your diet. With so many different types of soy foods available, there are endless (and delicious) options when you cook with soy.

Soy can be a main dish like broccoli tofu stir-fry, a light lunch dish like miso soup, or an ingredient in a mouth-watering dessert like Chocolate Raspberry Truffle Pie. It can also be a replacement food for meat and dairy products for people wanting a lower-fat, lower-cholesterol option. You can substitute soy ham for ham in your quiche recipe; replace the bologna, turkey, and cheese in your sandwiches with soy deli meats and cheeses; and make breakfast smoothies with chocolate or vanilla soy milk.

Cooking with soy is simple; it's a very adaptable food that blends well with other foods. You'll notice when cooking with soy foods like tofu and tempeh that they absorb the flavors of the other foods and seasonings in the dish. Soy's consistency and texture make it easy to add to a variety of dishes or eat on its own.

SOY SUBSTITUTIONS

Soy can also be used in cooking as a substitute for animal products that contain higher levels of saturated fat and cholesterol. Here are some of the most common soy substitutions:

YOU CAN REPLACE THIS:	WITH THIS:
Eggs	
1 egg	1 T soy flour plus 1 T water
1 egg	1 two-inch cube tofu
1 egg	2 ounces silken tofu

Cooking with Soy

YOU CAN REPLACE THIS:	WITH THIS:
Cheese and Cream	
1 cup ricotta cheese	1 cup firm tofu, mashed
Cream cheese	One-half of cream cheese can be replaced with silken tofu (or use soy cream cheese)
Sour cream	One-fourth of sour cream in dips can be replaced with silken tofu
Cream	One-half of cream in soups and sauces can be replaced with silken tofu
Margarine	
1 T margarine	¾ T vegetable oil*
1 c margarine	¾ c vegetable oil*
½ c margarine	⅓ c vegetable oil*
Fat	
Lard, butter, margarine	Equal amount of soy margarine
Chocolate	
1 oz. baking chocolate	3 T cocoa (powder) plus 1 T vegetable oil*

YOU CAN REPLACE THIS:	WITH THIS:
Milk	
Milk	Equal amount of soy milk
1 c buttermilk	1 c soy milk plus 2 T lemon juice
Flour	
2 T flour	1 T soy flour
Flour in baked goods	One-fourth of the flour in self-rising baked goods can be replaced with soy flour
Flour in quick breads	One-third of the flour in quick breads can be replaced with soy flour

*Wherever a substitution calls for vegetable oil, use soybean oil

(Adapted from: *1999 U.S. Soyfoods Directory;* Ohio Soybean Council; Minnesota Soybean Association)

HOW TO COOK WITH SOY

The thirty recipes in this chapter can be a starting place for you to experiment with different soy foods and learn how to cook with these foods. Some, obviously, have more soy in them than others. In addition to many tasty soy dishes that might be new to you, I've included several old favorites like lasagna and chili that can be made using soy meat alternatives to replace part or all of the meat.

All the recipes in this chapter were created and tested by Gail Simon, a professional chef and cooking instructor who has been using soy and whole foods in her cooking for more than twenty-five years. The nutritional analysis was conducted by Pacific Northwest Nutrition Services.

Here are a few tips to keep in mind when making these recipes:

- Recipes are guidelines. As you experiment with these dishes, feel free to add more (or use less) spice or salt to suit your taste.
- Dishes made with soy products may look different from their soyless counterparts. For example, quiche will look brown, not the yellow of quiche made with eggs.
- As you sample different soy products, like yogurt, soy sausage, and soy cheese, you might like different brands

better than others. Gail has listed her favorite brands in some of the recipes.

- Prep time includes activities like chopping, mixing, and sautéing, and cooking time refers to cooking or baking time.

How to Use the Nutritional Analysis

Please note that the nutritional values should be used as guides. Depending on the ingredients and brands of soy products you use, the values may vary. You'll notice that many of the recipes are low in saturated fat and most of the dishes have no, or very little, cholesterol.

The list below describes how the nutritional analysis was applied to the recipes:

- Optional ingredients were included in the analysis.
- Where choices were given for ingredients (for example, "use soy yogurt or soy ice cream"), the nutritional analysis includes only the first ingredient listed.
- The serving size used in soup and stew recipes was one cup.

- Dashes and pinches were analyzed as one-eighth teaspoon.
- A splash of wine was analyzed as one-half fluid ounce.
- 2 percent soy milk and full-fat flour was used in the analysis; you can use lower-fat versions when cooking.
- Any variations you make to these recipes will change the nutritional values.
- When cooking with tofu, drain the water and remove from container before slicing.
- The recommended serving sizes are based on the nutritional analysis for each recipe.

SOY RECIPES

Desserts and Snacks

You're not at your parents' dinner table anymore, so let's have dessert first! I admit I was skeptical about eating soy sweets, but as soon as I tasted Gail's creations, I had to swallow my words along with a second helping of pie.

Chocolate Raspberry Truffle Pie

Very rich, very delicious. Chocolate lovers won't be able to stop at one piece.

YIELD: 12 SERVINGS   PREP TIME: 15 MINUTES

12 ounces Mori-Nu silken tofu

3 cups milk chocolate or semisweet chocolate chips, melted over double boiler or in microwave

½ teaspoon almond extract

1 graham cracker crust, baked

½ cup raspberry jam, warmed

Fresh raspberries for garnish, in season

1. Combine tofu, melted chocolate chips, and almond extract in food processor. Blend until very smooth.

2. Pour mixture into the cooled pie crust.

3. Chill in the refrigerator for 2 hours or more.

4. To serve, spread jam over the pie and decorate with fresh berries.

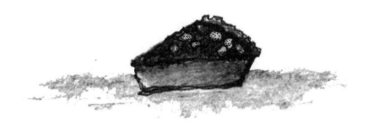

Per serving:							
CALORIES	TOTAL PROTEIN	SOY PROTEIN	TOTAL FAT	SATURATED FAT	CHOLESTEROL	SODIUM	FIBER
347	4 g	1 g	18 g	8 g	0 mg	125 mg	3 mg

Double Chocolate Soy Brownies

YIELD: EIGHT 2×4-INCH PIECES (SERVING SIZE: 1 BROWNIE)
PREP TIME: 15 MINUTES   COOKING TIME: 30 MINUTES

1½ cups chocolate chips
¼ cup butter
¾ cup white or brown sugar (or Florida Crystals brand
   dehydrated cane juice)
⅓ cup soy milk
1 extra-large egg
1 teaspoon vanilla extract
⅓ cup white flour
⅓ cup whole wheat pastry flour
⅓ cup unsweetened cocoa powder
1 teaspoon cinnamon
¾ teaspoon baking powder
pinch of salt

Cooking with Soy

1. Preheat oven to 350°F and grease an 8×8-inch pan.

2. Melt chocolate chips, butter, and sugar in a double boiler until smooth.

3. Combine milk, egg, and vanilla extract in a small bowl.

4. Mix dry ingredients in a large bowl.

5. Pour the milk mixture into the dry mixture and mix well.

6. Add the melted ingredients; stir until just combined. Do not overmix.

7. Pour into greased pan. Make sure batter fills pan evenly.

8. Bake for 30 minutes if using a glass pan, 35 minutes if using a metal pan.

9. Cool thoroughly before cutting. These brownies freeze well.

Per serving:

CALORIES	TOTAL PROTEIN	SOY PROTEIN	TOTAL FAT	SATURATED FAT	CHOLESTEROL	SODIUM	FIBER
384	6 g	0 g	19 g	10 g	44 mg	151 mg	4 mg

Fun Fruity Parfaits

Parfaits are perfect party desserts. Set up a dessert bar and everyone can make their favorite combinations. Kids love them, too.

SERVING SIZE: 1½ CUPS   PREP TIME: 5 MINUTES

soy yogurt or soy ice cream
fresh fruit or fruit spread
soy nuts
toasted coconut
carob or chocolate chips

1. Place a few spoonfuls of your favorite soy yogurt or soy ice cream in a tall parfait glass. Add a layer of sliced fruit or fruit spread.

2. Continue adding layers, alternating between yogurt and fruit. Top with soy nuts, toasted coconut, or carob or chocolate chips.

Cooking with Soy

VARIATIONS: Try these tasty parfait combos:

- Strawberry-flavored soy yogurt, sliced or crushed straw-berries and sliced bananas, toasted soy nuts.
- Vanilla soy ice cream, mango chunks, almond granola.
- Chocolate or carob soy ice cream, raspberry jam, coconut, and peanuts on top.
- Alternate three types of berry soy yogurt with toasted sun-flower seeds; slip thin, tart apple slices in around the edges.

Per serving:

CALORIES	TOTAL PROTEIN	SOY PROTEIN	TOTAL FAT	SATURATED FAT	CHOLESTEROL	SODIUM	FIBER
303	9 g	8 g	6 g	3 g	0 mg	186 mg	4 mg

Carrot Raisin Muffins with Soy Cream Drizzle

YIELD: 8 MUFFINS (SERVING SIZE: 1 MUFFIN)

PREP TIME: 10 MINUTES   COOKING TIME: 20 MINUTES

1 cup whole wheat pastry flour
⅔ cup unbleached white flour
⅓ cup soy flour
1 tablespoon baking powder
1 teaspoon cinnamon
¼ teaspoon nutmeg
⅛ teaspoon ginger
½ teaspoon salt
1 cup carrots, grated
½ cup raisins
1 egg or egg substitute
3 tablespoons honey
3 tablespoons oil
¾ cup soy milk

1. Preheat oven to 400°F.

2. Combine dry ingredients in a bowl, then add carrots and raisins.

3. Combine wet ingredients in a large mixing cup.

4. Add wet ingredients to dry ingredients and mix together with as few strokes as possible.

5. Pour batter into a well-greased muffin pan. Bake for 20 minutes.

Icing

2 tablespoons softened butter
½ cup soy cream cheese
¾ cup powdered sugar
½ teaspoon vanilla extract

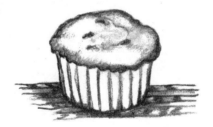

1. Cream the butter and cream cheese in a mixing bowl.
2. Add sugar and vanilla extract; mix until smooth.
3. Spread icing on the muffins after they have cooled.

Per serving:

CALORIES	TOTAL PROTEIN	SOY PROTEIN	TOTAL FAT	SATURATED FAT	CHOLESTEROL	SODIUM	FIBER
226	6 g	1 g	7 g	1 g	27 mg	313 mg	3 mg

Nut Butter Balls

Roasted soy nut butter gives these treats a hearty, nutty taste.

YIELD: 24 ONE-INCH BALLS (SERVING SIZE: 1 BALL)
PREP TIME: 15 MINUTES

½ cup soy nut butter
½ cup honey or rice syrup
¼ cup raisins

¼ cup grated dehydrated coconut

2 tablespoons raw sunflower seeds

2 teaspoons carob or unsweetened cocoa powder

½ cup coconut, sunflower seeds, crisp cereal, or
   mini-chocolate chips for coating

1. Combine first six ingredients in a cold bowl (use chilled ingredients).

2. Mix until ingredients blend to form a manageable ball.

3. Break off pieces and roll into balls about one inch in diameter.

4. Dip each ball in coating of your choice and roll it in your hands as you press the coating into the balls.

5. Store in refrigerator.

Per serving:

CALORIES	TOTAL PROTEIN	SOY PROTEIN	TOTAL FAT	SATURATED FAT	CHOLESTEROL	SODIUM	FIBER
73	0 g	0 g	5 g	1 g	0 mg	2 mg	0 mg

Breakfast and Brunch

Everyone knows that breakfast is the most important meal of
the day, but who has time to sit down and eat a nutritious meal?
Eating soy for breakfast is a great way to start the day with a
little bit of protein to get you through the morning. Whip up a
smoothie and you're out the door; pour soy milk over your cereal, use soy cream in your coffee, or toss a handful of soy nuts
on your soy yogurt and fruit.

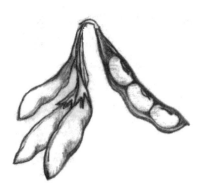

Breakfast Shakes and Smoothies

Start your day with a high-protein drink that includes a serving or two of fruit. Blend the shake or smoothie ingredients in a blender or food processor for several seconds or until it's smooth. Use chilled soy milk.

YIELD: 10 TO 12 OUNCES (SERVING SIZE: 10 OUNCES)
PREP TIME: 5 MINUTES

Melon Blondie

8 ounces soy milk
1 tablespoon vanilla-flavored soy protein powder
2 tablespoons frozen orange juice concentrate (or honey)
1 cup cubed cantaloupe (or peaches)

Per serving:

CALORIES	TOTAL PROTEIN	SOY PROTEIN	TOTAL FAT	SATURATED FAT	CHOLESTEROL	SODIUM	FIBER
230	18 g	15 g	5 g	1 g	0 mg	174 mg	5 mg

Chocolate Banana Date Smoothie

8 ounces chocolate soy milk
1 frozen banana, sliced
½ teaspoon cinnamon
¼ cup silken tofu
2 to 3 pitted dates*

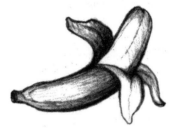

Per serving:

CALORIES	TOTAL PROTEIN	SOY PROTEIN	TOTAL FAT	SATURATED FAT	CHOLESTEROL	SODIUM	FIBER
666	28 g	27 g	21 g	0 g	0 mg	349 mg	8 mg

* If you don't like small pieces of date skin in your smoothie, use date pieces instead of pitted dates.

A Berry Good Shake

8 ounces vanilla soy milk
2 tablespoons frozen apple juice concentrate (or honey)
1 tablespoon soy protein powder, any flavor
1 cup frozen berries (or fresh, in season)

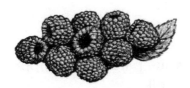

Per serving:

CALORIES	TOTAL PROTEIN	SOY PROTEIN	TOTAL FAT	SATURATED FAT	CHOLESTEROL	SODIUM	FIBER
343	17 g	15 g	6 g	0 g	0 mg	260 mg	8 mg

Brunch Quiche

This savory quiche is the perfect dish for Sunday brunch.

YIELD: 4 SERVINGS (SERVING SIZE: 1 PIECE)
PREP TIME: 15 MINUTES

COOKING TIME: 1 HOUR

3 garlic cloves, sliced
10 medium mushrooms, sliced
1 medium onion, sliced in half-moons
5 green onions (white part only), chopped
1 to 2 tablespoons oil
½ cup soy ham, diced
1 pound firm tofu
2 medium garlic cloves, smashed
2 tablespoons chopped green onion tops
3 tablespoons soy sauce
1 teaspoon thyme
1 pie crust, pricked with fork and prebaked for 12 minutes
    at 325°F.

1. Sauté the sliced garlic, mushrooms, onion, and green onions in oil for 5 minutes.

2. Add the soy ham and sauté for 2 minutes longer.

3. Combine the tofu, smashed garlic, green onion tops, soy sauce, and thyme in a blender or food processor.

4. Spoon the vegetable and soy ham mixture into the pie shell and spread the tofu mixture over it. Gently press the tofu mixture down into the vegetables.

5. Bake for 1 hour at 400°F until golden brown.

6. Cut with wet sharp knife.

Per serving:

CALORIES	TOTAL PROTEIN	SOY PROTEIN	TOTAL FAT	SATURATED FAT	CHOLESTEROL	SODIUM	FIBER
416	19 g	14 g	25 g	5 g	0 mg	1,152 mg	3 mg

Cinnamon Soy Pancakes

These moist pancakes are delicious topped with syrup, jam, or soy yogurt.

YIELD: 12 SMALL PANCAKES (SERVING SIZE: 1 PANCAKE)
PREP TIME: 5 MINUTES   COOKING TIME: 5 TO 10 MINUTES

1 cup white flour
¼ cup soy flour
¾ teaspoon cinnamon
pinch of salt
2 teaspoons sugar (or Florida Crystals brand
    dehydrated cane juice)
2 teaspoons baking powder
1 ¼ cups soy milk
2 teaspoons oil
½ teaspoon vanilla extract
cooking spray, oil, or butter

Cooking with Soy

1. Mix dry ingredients, then add wet ingredients. Stir mixture until combined.

2. Grease a frying pan or griddle with the cooking spray, oil, or butter, and heat.

3. Pour a small amount of batter onto the hot frying pan or griddle.

4. Cook very slowly on low heat so that the insides of the pancakes will be well cooked. (The soy flour makes these pancakes moister than regular pancakes.)

Per serving:

CALORIES	TOTAL PROTEIN	SOY PROTEIN	TOTAL FAT	SATURATED FAT	CHOLESTEROL	SODIUM	FIBER
64	2 g	1 g	2 g	0 g	0 mg	95 mg	1 mg

French Toast with Tofu Maple Cream

YIELD: 6 SERVINGS (SERVING SIZE: 1 SLICE TOAST WITH 1 TO 2 OUNCES CREAM)
PREP TIME: 10 MINUTES   COOKING TIME: 5 TO 10 MINUTES

French Toast

cooking spray, oil, or butter
3 eggs, beaten
1 teaspoon vanilla or maple extract
¾ cup soy milk
6 slices whole-grain bread

1. Grease a frying pan or griddle with the cooking spray, oil, or butter, and heat to medium hot.

2. Combine eggs, vanilla or maple extract, and soy milk in a wide bowl.

3. Dip bread into mixture, one slice at a time, and let excess batter drip off.

4. Fry the bread at medium heat until golden brown on each side.

Tofu Maple Cream

YIELD: 1½ CUPS   PREP TIME: 5 MINUTES

12.3-ounce box silken tofu
3 tablespoons maple syrup
½ teaspoon cinnamon
½ teaspoon vanilla extract

1. Combine all ingredients in blender or food processor until smooth and creamy.

2. Serve over warm French toast or on the side as a dipping sauce.

Per serving:

CALORIES	TOTAL PROTEIN	SOY PROTEIN	TOTAL FAT	SATURATED FAT	CHOLESTEROL	SODIUM	FIBER
175	11 g	4 g	6 g	1 g	106 mg	209 mg	4 mg

Tofu Scramble with Fresh Herbs

*Filled with vegetables and seasoned with fresh herbs,
this colorful scramble will quickly become a favorite
on your breakfast and brunch menus.*

YIELD: 3 SERVINGS (SERVING SIZE: 1 CUP)

PREP TIME: 10 MINUTES   COOKING TIME: 10 MINUTES

2 tablespoons oil

⅓ cup red bell pepper, diced

⅓ cup red or yellow onion, diced

½ cup carrot or zucchini, grated or diced

¼ cup shallots, minced (optional)

1 pound firm tofu, crumbled

½ teaspoon turmeric, for color

½ cup loosely packed chopped herbs, such as Italian
   parsley, basil, or dill

2 garlic cloves, minced or pressed

salt or soy sauce to taste

Cooking with Soy

1. In a hot skillet, heat the oil.

2. Sauté the vegetables for 5 minutes, until the onion begins to brown.

3. Add tofu, turmeric, herbs, garlic, and salt or soy sauce; mix well.

4. Cook until the vegetables are tender, adding drops of water to the mixture if it sticks to the pan.

5. Serve with soy sausages or tempeh bacon.

Per serving:

CALORIES	TOTAL PROTEIN	SOY PROTEIN	TOTAL FAT	SATURATED FAT	CHOLESTEROL	SODIUM	FIBER
234	14 g	12 g	16 g	2 g	0 mg	28 mg	2 mg

Lunch

Break out of your lunchtime rut with these tasty soups, salads, and sandwiches.

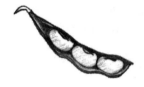

Tusc-Asian Bean Soup with Garlic and Sage

Two white beans from different continents team up in this simple and delicious soup. Serve with a loaf of crusty bread.

YIELD: 2 QUARTS (SERVING SIZE: 1 CUP)

PREP TIME: 10 MINUTES   COOKING TIME: 15 MINUTES

Cooking with Soy

1 small onion, coarsely chopped
1 rib celery, coarsely chopped
4 tablespoons olive oil
5 garlic cloves, minced
about 9 fresh sage leaves, slivered
1 can cannellini beans
1 can yellow soybeans
2 cups stock, water, or bean liquid (or combination)
1 cup loosely packed torn spinach leaves
salt and pepper to taste
1 cup cooked orzo pasta (½ cup uncooked)
splash of balsamic or red-wine vinegar for each diner

1. Sauté onion and celery in oil on low heat for 5 minutes.

2. Add garlic and sage;* sauté for 3 more minutes. Do not brown the garlic.

3. Add beans, stock (or other liquid), spinach, salt, and pepper. Bring to a boil.

*If you cannot get fresh sage leaves, simply sauté the garlic alone and add ½ teaspoon dried sage to the pot after the liquid has been added.

4. Reduce to simmer and cook for 5 minutes.

5. Puree the soup in a blender or food processor to an almost smooth texture.

6. Add the cooked orzo and serve.

7. Provide vinegar for garnish.

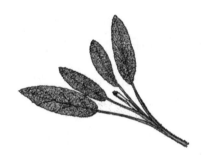

Per serving:							
CALORIES	TOTAL PROTEIN	SOY PROTEIN	TOTAL FAT	SATURATED FAT	CHOLESTEROL	SODIUM	FIBER
243	12 g	7 g	12 g	2 g	17 mg	356 mg	5 mg

Light and Fresh
Miso Soup

Traditionally, miso soup is made with dashi, a broth made of kombu seaweed and dried fish flakes. This quick and easy variation uses vegetable stock or bouillon cubes.

YIELD: 1 QUART (SERVING SIZE: 1 CUP)

PREP TIME: 10 MINUTES   COOKING TIME: 10 MINUTES

1 cup sliced green onions (white parts only)
2 garlic cloves, minced
1 teaspoon toasted sesame oil
1-inch piece of ginger root, grated and squeezed
   for its juice
1 cup firm tofu, cut in very small cubes
4 cups hot stock, or 4 cups mixture of water and stock
4 teaspoons blond (white), red, or yellow miso paste

1. In a saucepan, sauté the white parts of the green onion and the garlic in the sesame oil on low heat for 2 minutes.

2. Add the rest of the ingredients, except the miso paste, and bring to a boil.

3. Take a ladle of liquid from the pot and place it in a small bowl. Dissolve the miso in the liquid.

4. Reduce the heat and gently simmer the soup. Add the miso solution.

5. Increase the heat for a few minutes without bringing the soup to a boil. (Boiling at this stage will make the soup taste bitter.) Serve with a side dish of rice or noodles. Optional: Chop up the tops of green onions and use them as garnish.

Per serving:

CALORIES	TOTAL PROTEIN	SOY PROTEIN	TOTAL FAT	SATURATED FAT	CHOLESTEROL	SODIUM	FIBER
101	8 g	6 g	5 g	1 g	0 mg	1,218 mg	1 mg

Warm Pasta Salad with Basil Tofu Dressing

YIELD: 6 SERVINGS (SERVING SIZE: 1 CUP)

PREP TIME: 15 MINUTES   COOKING TIME: 15 MINUTES

2 tablespoons olive oil
5 garlic cloves, sliced
1 medium zucchini, cut into bite-size pieces
1 medium ripe tomato, cut into bite-size pieces
½ cup loosely packed basil leaves, slivered
½ pound macaroni, such as penne or shells,
   cooked and well drained
1 tablespoon red wine vinegar
½ pound soft or silken tofu, drained
3 tablespoons fresh lemon juice
1 teaspoon lemon zest from organic lemon
salt and black pepper to taste

1. In a hot frying pan, heat the olive oil; sauté the garlic and zucchini for 2 to 3 minutes on medium heat.

2. Add tomato and basil and cook for one minute while stirring.

3. Add the contents of the frying pan to the cooked macaroni.

4. Pour the vinegar into the hot pan and deglaze, scraping up any remaining bits of food. Pour this liquid over the pasta and mix it in.

5. Combine the tofu, lemon juice and zest, salt, and pepper in a blender or food processor. Mix until smooth.

6. Add this mixture to the salad. Eat warm or chilled.

VARIATIONS: Add one or more of the following to the salad:

½ cup olives
½ cup diced sun-dried tomatoes in olive oil
½ cup toasted pine nuts or walnut pieces

Per serving:							
CALORIES	TOTAL PROTEIN	SOY PROTEIN	TOTAL FAT	SATURATED FAT	CHOLESTEROL	SODIUM	FIBER
75	2 g	2 g	6 g	1 g	0 mg	54 mg	1 mg

Tempting Tempeh "Turkey" Salad with Poppy Seed Dressing

Replace part or all of the turkey in this summer salad with tempeh for a new twist on an old favorite. A perfect picnic dish.

Yield: about 3 cups (serving size: 1 cup)   Prep time: 20 minutes

8-ounce block tempeh, cut into ½-inch cubes
   or use
4 ounces tempeh, cut into ½-inch cubes, and 4 ounces
   cooked, diced turkey meat
vegetable broth
1 small tart crisp apple, diced into ½-inch cubes;
   or ⅔ cup grapes, halved
1 large rib celery, thinly sliced
⅓ cup minced sweet yellow or red onion

1. Simmer the tempeh pieces for 5 minutes in vegetable broth (use just enough broth to cover the pieces). This process makes the tempeh easier to digest.

2. Combine all the ingredients in a large bowl.

3. Toss gently with ½ cup Poppy Seed Dressing (see recipe on page 143). Serve chilled.

VARIATIONS: Try these serving ideas:

- Arrange salad in a lettuce cup and serve on decorative plates.
- Serve salad in a tomato cup. Slice a firm, ripe tomato from top to bottom, cutting only three-fourths of the way down. Make a similar cut perpendicular to the first to make four sections. Gently pull the sections back to make a flower in the center of the tomato. Add a scoop of salad into the tomato and place on a plate covered with crisp lettuce.

Per serving:

CALORIES	TOTAL PROTEIN	SOY PROTEIN	TOTAL FAT	SATURATED FAT	CHOLESTEROL	SODIUM	FIBER
261	13 g	13 g	18 g	2 g	8 mg	101 mg	4 mg

Tofu Guacamole Wraps

A wrap is a sandwich made with a flat bread, like a wheat tortilla, chapati, tanoor, or lefse. Add your favorite filling— grilled vegetables, egg salad, hummus, or this tofu guacamole, and roll it up.

YIELD: FILLING FOR 2 WRAPS (SERVING SIZE: 1 WRAP)
PREP TIME: 10 MINUTES

1 small ripe avocado or half of a larger variety
¼ cup soft or firm tofu
1 to 2 tablespoons fresh lime or lemon juice
2 tablespoons tomato salsa
1 tablespoon minced onion or green onion
minced jalapeno or hot sauce to taste (optional)
1 tablespoon Garlic Miso Spread (see recipe on page 139)
2 flat breads
2 small, soft lettuce leaves, washed and dried
4 slices ripe tomato
handful of soy sprouts (or other sprouts)

———

1. In a small bowl mash the first six ingredients to make the tofu guacamole.

2. Smooth miso spread on the inside of the bread. Add a lettuce leaf, then top lettuce with tofu guacamole, sliced tomato, and sprouts. Make sure that the ingredients are spread evenly across the bread.

3. Roll bread carefully.

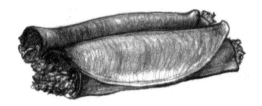

Per serving:

CALORIES	TOTAL PROTEIN	SOY PROTEIN	TOTAL FAT	SATURATED FAT	CHOLESTEROL	SODIUM	FIBER
243	7 g	3 g	12 g	2 g	0 mg	225 mg	5 mg

Italian Sausage Hoagies with Peppers and Onions

This sandwich brings me back to New York City's Italian street festivals, where the scents of garlic and fried onions filled the air.

YIELD: FILLING FOR 4 SANDWICHES (SERVING SIZE: 1 SANDWICH)
PREP AND COOKING TIME: 15 MINUTES

2 tablespoons olive oil

1 medium red or green bell pepper, cut in slivers

1 large onion, cut in thin half-moons

3 to 4 garlic cloves, sliced

5 Lightlife Lean Links Italian sausages, each cut into 4 even pieces

mayonnaise (or soy mayonnaise) or thick garlic salad dressing

4 (6-inch-length) Italian or French rolls or 4 pita pockets

1. Heat oil in a large frying pan.

2. Sauté pepper and onion on medium heat for 10 minutes, stirring now and then.

3. Add garlic and sausage; cook for 5 more minutes or until sausage is browned.

4. Spread mayonnaise or dressing on rolls or pita and fill with equal portions of the vegetable-sausage mixture.

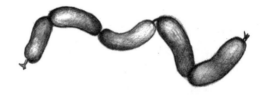

Per serving:							
CALORIES	TOTAL PROTEIN	SOY PROTEIN	TOTAL FAT	SATURATED FAT	CHOLESTEROL	SODIUM	FIBER
394	12 g	5 g	22 g	3 g	8 mg	565 mg	3 mg

Spicy Soba Noodles with Soy Nuts

YIELD: 2 TO 4 SERVINGS

PREP TIME: 10 MINUTES   COOKING TIME: 10 TO 15 MINUTES

¼ cup soy nut butter

3 tablespoons soy sauce

1 to 3 tablespoons water

2½ tablespoons rice vinegar

1 tablespoon toasted sesame oil

1 tablespoon honey

2 small garlic cloves

1 green onion, sliced

½ teaspoon ground ginger or 1 teaspoon juice from fresh
   ginger

few pinches cayenne pepper, to taste

8 ounces cooked long noodles (Japanese soba or Chinese
   noodles are best, but spaghetti will work just fine)

roasted soy nuts for garnish (optional)

1. Combine all ingredients except noodles and nuts in blender or processor and mix until smooth. Adjust liquid as needed and spice to taste. This dressing needs to be thin enough to coat the noodles yet thick enough to stick to them.

2. Mix dressing thoroughly into cooked, warm noodles.

3. Garnish with soy nuts if desired. Best served chilled or at room temperature.

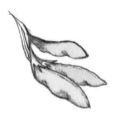

Per serving:

CALORIES	TOTAL PROTEIN	SOY PROTEIN	TOTAL FAT	SATURATED FAT	CHOLESTEROL	SODIUM	FIBER
441	8 g	2 g	30 g	5 g	0 mg	1,623 mg	1 mg

Salad Dressings and Spreads

These dressings and spreads are rich and fresh in flavor, low in fat and cholesterol. The serving size for all the dressings and spreads is one ounce.

Garlic Miso Spread

YIELD: ¾ CUP   PREP TIME: 10 MINUTES

2 level tablespoons dark-type miso
3 level tablespoons unsalted soy nut butter
1 garlic clove, pressed
1 tablespoon slivered scallion greens or chives
squirt of lemon juice (optional)
¼ teaspoon fresh ginger root, finely minced or grated
    and squeezed for its juice (optional)
¼ cup water

1. Place all the ingredients, including the optional ingredients, if desired, except the water in a small bowl.

2. Add water and stir until you have a smooth spread, with a consistency similar to whipped cream cheese. (You may need to use a bit more than ¼ cup of water.)

3. Taste. If too salty, add 1 more teaspoon soy nut butter.

4. Serve spread on flat bread, crackers, or rice cakes, topped with sprouts or cheese. Also delicious on warm steamed vegetables, mixed into a bowl of hot rice, or thinly spread in the cavity of fresh celery.

5. Store in refrigerator in a tightly sealed container. Will stay fresh for 2 to 3 weeks.

Per serving:

CALORIES	TOTAL PROTEIN	SOY PROTEIN	TOTAL FAT	SATURATED FAT	CHOLESTEROL	SODIUM	FIBER
63	1 g	0 g	6 g	1 g	0 mg	211 mg	0 mg

Honey Mustard Dressing

YIELD: 1 CUP   PREP TIME: 5 MINUTES

1 tablespoon plus 1 teaspoon Dijon mustard
2 tablespoons plus 2 teaspoons honey
2 tablespoons plus 2 teaspoons apple cider vinegar
½ cup canola oil
¾ cup plain or vanilla soy milk

Combine all ingredients and shake or mix until well blended.

Per serving:

CALORIES	TOTAL PROTEIN	SOY PROTEIN	TOTAL FAT	SATURATED FAT	CHOLESTEROL	SODIUM	FIBER
153	1 g	0 g	14 g	1 g	0 mg	18 mg	0 mg

Creamy Italian Dressing

YIELD: 1 CUP

PREP TIME: 7 MINUTES

⅓ cup silken tofu
¼ cup red- or white-wine vinegar
2 tablespoons olive oil
1 tablespoon vegetable stock or water
1 teaspoon dried basil
1 teaspoon dried oregano
1 teaspoon dried thyme
1 small or medium garlic clove, smashed
salt and pepper to taste

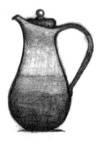

Place all ingredients in a blender or food processor and blend until smooth and creamy. This dressing goes with the Protein Power Dinner Salad (see page 145).

Per serving:							
CALORIES	TOTAL PROTEIN	SOY PROTEIN	TOTAL FAT	SATURATED FAT	CHOLESTEROL	SODIUM	FIBER
44	1 g	0 g	4 g	0 g	0 mg	133 mg	0 mg

Poppy Seed Dressing

YIELD: ½ CUP   PREP TIME: 5 MINUTES

3 tablespoons mayonnaise of your choice
2 tablespoons soy or dairy yogurt, plain or vanilla flavored
2 tablespoons orange juice (fresh squeezed is best)
½ teaspoon honey
1 teaspoon poppy seeds

Combine all ingredients in a bowl and mix until well blended. This dressing goes with Tempting Tempeh "Turkey" Salad (see page 131).

Per serving:							
CALORIES	TOTAL PROTEIN	SOY PROTEIN	TOTAL FAT	SATURATED FAT	CHOLESTEROL	SODIUM	FIBER
92	1 g	0 g	9 g	1 g	6 mg	62 mg	0 mg

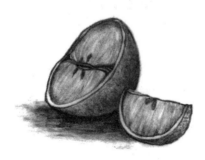

Dinner

You don't have to be a whiz at Asian cooking to make delicious soy dishes.

Protein Power Dinner Salad

Turn an ordinary side salad into a protein-packed meal.

YIELD: 4 SERVINGS (SERVING SIZE: 2 CUPS)
PREP TIME: 10 MINUTES (PLUS MARINATING TIME)

1 cup canned black or white soybeans
1 cup fresh green soybeans (edamame), cooked*
4 cups packed assorted salad greens, washed, dried, and torn
½ cup chopped fresh herbs, such as basil or parsley
2 cups assorted vegetables and herbs, such as cucumber, radish, tomato, onion, carrots, or celery

*See page 79 for more information about edamame.

1. Earlier in the day or even the night before, marinate the beans in ½ cup Creamy Italian Dressing (see page 142) and refrigerate.

2. Toss the salad greens with the herbs in a large bowl.

3. Sprinkle the other vegetables over the greens.

4. Spoon the marinated beans in a mound in the center of the salad.

5. Drizzle the marinade and as much additional dressing as you like over the salad.

6. Toss just before serving.

Per serving:

CALORIES	TOTAL PROTEIN	SOY PROTEIN	TOTAL FAT	SATURATED FAT	CHOLESTEROL	SODIUM	FIBER
416	35 g	33 g	5 g	1 g	0 mg	57 mg	10 mg

Vegetarian Chili over Mashed Potatoes

Nothing will warm you up like hot chili served over a favorite comfort food—mashed potatoes. Stretch this recipe by adding more beans, corn, and sauce.

YIELD: 4 SERVINGS (SERVING SIZE: 1½ TO 2 CUPS OF CHILI
OVER ½ CUP MASHED POTATOES)

PREP TIME: 10 MINUTES   COOKING TIME: 20 MINUTES

1 cup diced onion in small pieces
1 cup diced bell pepper in small pieces
3 garlic cloves, minced
½ cup textured soy protein soaked in ½ cup stock or water
1 can white soybeans, drained
1 can black soybeans or black beans, drained
1 cup cut corn
2½ cups thick tomato sauce
2 teaspoons chili powder
1 teaspoon oregano

cayenne pepper or minced jalapeno pepper to taste
handful of cilantro (Chinese parsley) leaves, chopped
fluffy mashed potatoes*

1. Sauté onion and bell pepper in a large pot for 5 to 6 minutes.

2. Add everything else except the cilantro and mashed potatoes.

3. Bring to a boil, then lower heat immediately to a gentle simmer. Cover and cook for at least 15 minutes.

4. Stir in cilantro leaves during the last 5 minutes of cooking.

5. Serve hot over a dollop of mashed potatoes.

Per serving:							
CALORIES	TOTAL PROTEIN	SOY PROTEIN	TOTAL FAT	SATURATED FAT	CHOLESTEROL	SODIUM	FIBER
872	67 g	60 g	29 g	3 g	2 mg	1,392 mg	16 mg

*The nutritional analysis is based on mashed potatoes made with milk, with a serving size equal to ½ cup.

Erika's Zucchini and Garlic Pizza

1 tablespoon olive oil

½ cup onion, in thin half-moon slices

½ cup slivered fresh red bell pepper, or sliced roasted
   red pepper

1 small zucchini, in very thin slices

3 garlic cloves, sliced

1 cup soy meats: pepperoni, crumbled sausage, or ham

½ cup tomato-based pizza sauce, or pesto sauce

1 large pizza crust

1 ½ cups soy or dairy mozzarella cheese

2 to 3 tablespoons soy or dairy Parmesan cheese

1. Heat oil in skillet.

2. Sauté onion, bell pepper (roasted red pepper does not need to be sautéed), zucchini, garlic, and soy meat for about 5 minutes, until vegetables are tender.

3. Spread tomato or pesto sauce on pizza crust.

4. Arrange sautéed vegetable-meat mixture on top of sauce.

5. Top crust with cheeses.

6. Bake at 400°F for about 15 minutes, being careful not to brown the soy cheeses. (See page 85 for more information on cooking with soy cheese.)

Per serving:

CALORIES	TOTAL PROTEIN	SOY PROTEIN	TOTAL FAT	SATURATED FAT	CHOLESTEROL	SODIUM	FIBER
302	19 g	15 g	15 g	2 g	0 mg	770 mg	4 mg

Spinach Lasagna

YIELD: 12 PIECES (SERVING SIZE: 1 PIECE)

PREP TIME: 30 MINUTES   COOKING TIME: 1½ HOURS

6 cups flavorful tomato sauce

10-ounce box spinach, defrosted, squeezed well, and
  chopped

1 package Yves Veggie Ground Round or Lightlife Gimme
  Lean, crumbled and browned in olive oil*

1½ pounds soft tofu, drained

½ cup fresh basil

2 teaspoons dried oregano

¼ teaspoon ground pepper

3 to 4 large garlic cloves, smashed

3 cups grated soy mozzarella

½ cup soy Parmesan cheese

10 lasagna noodles, cooked (but still firm) and rinsed well

*Read cooking instructions on package. Some soy ground round doesn't need to be browned.

1. In a large bowl, combine the tomato sauce, spinach, and soy crumble.

2. In blender or food processor, combine the tofu, basil, oregano, pepper, and garlic.

3. Combine the two cheeses in a bowl.

4. Preheat oven to 375°F.

5. Pour a small amount of sauce mixture on the bottom of an 8×11-inch glass or ceramic baking dish (enough to coat dish).

6. Place 4 lasagna noodles on the bottom of the baking dish.

7. Spread one-third of the tofu mixture evenly over the noodles.

8. Spoon one-third of the sauce mixture over tofu mixture, spreading it evenly.

9. Sprinkle a couple of tablespoons of cheese mixture over the sauce.

10. Repeat steps 6 to 9, using 3 noodles per layer and ending with the sauce mixture.

11. Bake covered for 1 hour and 15 minutes.

12. Uncover, sprinkle remaining cheese mixture over the top, and bake uncovered for 15 more minutes.

13. Let lasagna cool for 10 minutes before cutting.

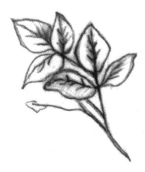

Per serving:							
CALORIES	TOTAL PROTEIN	SOY PROTEIN	TOTAL FAT	SATURATED FAT	CHOLESTEROL	SODIUM	FIBER
443	29 g	13 g	14 g	3 g	26 mg	953 mg	5 mg

Stuffed Bell Peppers

*A colorful and festive dish, these peppers taste great stuffed
with veggie ground round, rice, and classic seasonings.
You won't miss the meat!*

Yield: 6 medium peppers (serving size: 2 pepper halves)
Prep time: 20 minutes   Cooking time: 1 hour

6 medium bell peppers, round and wide for stuffing
14-ounce package Yves Veggie Ground Round
⅔ cup long-grain uncooked white rice or same amount of
   brown rice, cooked halfway through
1 carrot, grated
⅓ cup sunflower seeds
½ cup raisins
2 tablespoons chopped fresh parsley
4 garlic cloves, pressed or minced
2 teaspoons dried basil
1 teaspoon dried thyme
salt and pepper to taste
5 cups tomato sauce mixed with 1 ½ cups stock or water

1. Carefully cut peppers in half, from top to bottom, and re-move stem, seeds, and membrane. Place peppers in a pot of boiling water, cover, and cook for 3 minutes. Remove peppers from water and set aside.

2. In a large bowl, combine all the remaining ingredients except the tomato sauce. Mix in 1 cup of tomato sauce to moisten mixture.

3. Fill the pepper shells with the mixture and lay pepper halves on their backs in a baking dish.

4. Pour a generous amount of sauce over each pepper to keep it moist during baking, and pour the remaining sauce into the baking dish.

5. Bake tightly covered for 1 hour at 400°F.

VARIATIONS: You may omit the sunflower seeds and raisins and add an extra grated carrot or a small chopped zucchini instead. If you like your pepper shells firm, eliminate the blanching step.

Per serving:

CALORIES	TOTAL PROTEIN	SOY PROTEIN	TOTAL FAT	SATURATED FAT	CHOLESTEROL	SODIUM	FIBER
258	17 g	10 g	5 g	0 g	0 mg	1,550 mg	7 mg

Tofu and Broccoli with Black Bean Sauce

A stir-fry for all seasons that you can serve with rice or noodles.
You can also add shrimp or chunks of grilled halibut.
Quick and easy dinner idea for any season.

YIELD: 4 SERVINGS (SERVING SIZE: 1 CUP)

PREP TIME: 15 MINUTES   COOKING TIME: 15 MINUTES

2 teaspoons canola oil
1 teaspoon toasted sesame oil
1 pound firm tofu, cubed
3 garlic cloves, slivered
1 bunch broccoli, cut into florets and blanched
1 tablespoon Chinese black bean sauce*

*Sun Luck or Lee Kum Kee brands are available in most supermarkets.

Cooking with Soy

1. Heat oils in large frying pan.

2. Sauté tofu and garlic for 5 minutes.

3. Add blanched broccoli and black bean sauce.

4. Stir well and heat all the way through. Add a few drops of water if too thick.

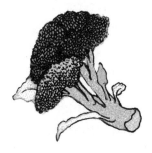

Per serving:

CALORIES	TOTAL PROTEIN	SOY PROTEIN	TOTAL FAT	SATURATED FAT	CHOLESTEROL	SODIUM	FIBER
140	11 g	9 g	9 g	1 g	0 mg	83 mg	2 mg

Curried Red Lentil Stew with Tempeh

YIELD: 2 QUARTS (SERVING SIZE: 1 CUP)

PREP TIME: 10 MINUTES   COOKING TIME: 30 MINUTES

2 tablespoons oil

8-ounce block of White Wave or Turtle Island brand
    tempeh, cut in 1-inch cubes

1 teaspoon curry powder

1 teaspoon ground cumin

½ teaspoon salt

1 cup celery, cut in 1-inch chunks

1 cup onions, cut in 1-inch chunks

1 cup carrots, cut in 1-inch chunks

1 cup potatoes, cut in 1-inch chunks

5 garlic cloves, chopped

1 cup split red lentils

4 cups vegetable or chicken stock, or water

½ cup canned diced tomatoes

handful cilantro or parsley, chopped, for garnish

Cooking with Soy

1. Heat oil in soup pot. Add tempeh and brown on low heat for 5 minutes, turning tempeh with a spatula to brown all sides.

2. Add seasonings; stir and cook for 1 more minute.

3. Add everything else except the cilantro and bring stew to a boil.

4. Reduce to a simmer, cover, and cook for 20 minutes.

5. Check vegetables for tenderness. Stir in cilantro or parsley. Serve.

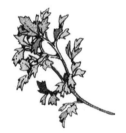

Per serving:

CALORIES	TOTAL PROTEIN	SOY PROTEIN	TOTAL FAT	SATURATED FAT	CHOLESTEROL	SODIUM	FIBER
388	14 g	6 g	6 g	1 g	0 mg	6,349 mg	11 mg

Notes

Anderson, J. W., M. B. Johnstone, and M. E. Cook-Newell, "Meta-analysis of the Effects of Soy Protein Intake on Serum Lipids," *New England Journal of Medicine* 333, no. 5 (1995): 276–82.

Arjmandi, H. G. et al., "Dietary Soybean Protein Prevents Bone Loss in an Ovariectomised Rat Model of Osteoporosis," *Journal of Nutrition* 126 (1996): 161–67.

Atkins, F. M., and E. Auld, "Food Allergy Basics: What Clinicians Should Know," *Nutrition and the MD* 19, no. 4 (1993): 1–5.

Barnes, S. et al., "Soybeans Inhibit Mammary Tumors in Models of Breast Cancer," *Mutagens and Carcinogens in the Diet* (New York: Wiley-Liss, 1990), 239–53.

Bryan, F. R., *Henry's Lieutenants* (Detroit: Wayne State University Press, 1993).

Carroll, K. K., "Review of Clinical Studies on Cholesterol-Lowering Response to Soy Protein," *Journal of the American Dietetic Association* 91 (1991): 820–27.

Notes

Coward, L. et al., "Genistein, Daidzein, and Their Glycoside Conjugates: Antitumor Isoflavones in Soybean Foods from American and Asian Diets," *Journal of Agricultural Food Chemistry* 41 (1993): 1961–67.

Dunn, J. E., "Cancer Epidemiology in Populations of the United States with Emphasis on Hawaii, California, and Japan," *Cancer Research* 35, no. 11 (1975): 3240–45.

Greenberg, P., *The Whole Soy Cookbook* (New York: Three Rivers Press, 1998).

Hasler, C., "Soy and Human Health," Stratsoy Web site, University of Illinois (www.ag.uiuc.edu/~stratsoy/expert/askhealth.html).

Helmuth, L., "Nutritionists Debate Soy's Health Benefits," *Science News* 155, no. 17 (April 24, 1999): 262(1).

Hu, J. et al., "Diet and Cancer of the Colon and Rectum: A Case-Control Study in China," *International Journal of Epidemiology* 20 (1991): 362–67.

Kim, H., H. Xia, L. Lin, and J. Gewin, "Attenuation of Neurodegeneration Markers by Dietary Soy," *BioFactors* (2000).

Knight, D. C., and J. A. Eden, "A Review of the Clinical Effects of Phytoestrogens," *American Journal of Obstetrics and Gynecology* 87, no. 5 (1996): 897–904.

Kolonel, L. N., "Variability in Diet and Its Relation to Risk in Ethnic and Migrant Groups," *Basic Life Science* 43 (1998): 129–35.

Lee, H. P. et al., "Dietary Effects on Breast-Cancer Risk in Singapore," *Lancet* 337, no. 8751 (1991): 1197–1200.

Notes

Liebman, B., "The Soy Story," *Nutrition Action Healthletter* 25, no. 7 (September 1998): 1(6).

Lo, G. S. et al., "Soy Fiber Improves Lipid and Carbohydrate Metabolism in Primary Hyperlipidemic Subjects," *Atherosclerosis* 62 (1986): 239–48.

Lock, M., "Menopause in Cultural Context," *Experimental Gerontology* 29, no. 3–4 (1994): 307–17.

Mensink, R. P., and M. B. Katan, "Effect of Dietary Fatty Acids on Serum Lipids and Lipoproteins: A Meta-analysis of Twenty-seven Trials," *Arteriosclerosis, Thrombosis, and Vascular Biology* 12 (1992): 911–19.

Messina, M. et al., "Soy Intake and Cancer Risk: A Review of the In Vitro and In Vivo Data," *Nutrition and Cancer* 21 (1994): 113–31.

Messina, M., and S. Barnes, "The Role of Soy Products in Reducing Risk of Cancer," *Journal of the National Cancer Institute* 83, no. 8 (1991): 541–46.

Messina, M., and V. Messina, "Soyfoods & Allergies," "Soyfoods & Bone Health," "Soyfoods & Cancer," "Soyfoods & Diabetes," "Soyfoods & Heart Disease," "Soyfoods & Iron," "Soyfoods & Isoflavones," "Soyfoods & Kidney Health," "Soyfoods & Nutrients," "Soyfoods & Protein," "Soyfoods & Women's Health," *Soy Facts* (Indiana Soybean Board).

———, *Soyfood for Thought* (Indiana Soybean Board).

Messina, M., V. Messina, and K. D. R. Setchell, *The Simple Soybean and Your Health* (Garden City Park, N.Y.: Avery Publishing Group, 1994).

Notes

Murkies, A. L. et al., "Dietary Flour Supplementation Decreases Post-menopausal Hot Flushes: Effect of Soy and Wheat," *Maturitas* 21, no. 3 (1995): 189–95.

Napier, K., "Taking Soy to Heart," *Harvard Health Letter* 21 (November 1995): 1(2).

Nomura, A. et al., "Breast Cancer and Diet among the Japanese in Hawaii," *American Journal of Clinical Nutrition* 31, no. 11 (1978): 2020–25.

Pan, Y., M. A. Anthony, S. Watson, and T. B. Clarkson, "Soy Phytoestrogens Improve Radial Arm Maze Performance in Ovariectomized Retired Breeder Rats and Do Not Attentuate Benefits of 17-beta Estradiol Treatment," *Menopause* (2000).

Potter, S. M. et al., "Depression of Plasma Cholesterol in Men by Consumption of Baked Products Containing Soy Protein," *American Journal of Clinical Nutrition* 58, no. 4 (1993): 501–6.

Sears, B., *The Soy Zone* (New York: Regan Books, 2000).

Severson, R. K. et al., "A Prospective Study of Demographics, Diet, and Prostate Cancer among Men of Japanese Ancestry in Hawaii," *Cancer Research* 49 (1989): 1857–60.

Singh, M., E. M. Meyer, W. J. Millard, and J. W. Simpkins, "Ovarian Steroid Deprivation Results in a Reversible Learning Impairment and Compromised Cholinergic Function in Female Sprague-Dawley Rats," *Brain Research* 644 (1994): 305–12.

Stevens, J. A., and R. H. Stevens, eds., *1999 U.S. Soyfoods Directory* (Indianapolis: Stevens and Associates, Inc., 1999).

Sullivan, C., and K. Rhodes, *Simply Soy: A Variety of Choices* (Frankenmuth: Michigan Soybean Promotion Committee).

Notes

Watanabe, Y. et al., "A Case-Control Study of Cancer of the Rectum and the Colon," *Nippon Shokakibyo Gakkai Zasshi* 81 (1984): 185–94.

Winter, R., *Super Soy* (New York: Crown Trade Paperbacks, 1996).

Cancer Facts and Figures, American Cancer Society Web site (www.cancer.org).

Creative Cooking with Soy (Columbus: Ohio Soybean Council).

"FDA Approves Health Claim for Soy Protein," *Energy Times* (January 2000): 12.

The 5,000-Year-Old Secret for Delicious and Nutritious Meals (St. Louis: United Soybean Board).

Guide to Using the New Soy Health Claim (Decatur, Ill.: Archer Daniels Midland).

"Healthful Options for Fat in the Diet," "Incorporating Optimal Levels of Protein in the Diet," "The Healthful, Balanced Nutrient," "Advancements in Plant Biotechnology," "Discovering the Health Benefits of Isoflavones," "Preventing and Treating Heart Disease," "Women's Health and Disease Prevention," "Understanding Allergies and Dietary Options," "Preventing and Treating Cancer," and "Preventing and Treating Diabetes and Kidney Disease," *Soy and Health Fact Sheets* (St. Louis: United Soybean Board).

How a 5,000-Year-Old Bean Is Making America Healthier (St. Louis: United Soybean Board, 1998).

"Second International Symposium on the Role of Soy in Preventing and Treating Chronic Disease," 1997 Web site, Indiana Soybean Board (www.soyfoods.com/symposium).

Notes

Soybean Oil Gives Products the One Thing Other Oils Can't (St. Louis: United Soybean Board).

Soybeans: How a Little Bean Becomes an Ingredient in Thousands of Products (St. Louis: United Soybean Board).

Soy Facts (Columbus: Ohio Soybean Council, 1998).

Soy Foods fact sheets (Washington, D.C.: Soyfoods Association of North America).

Soy Protein and Health: Discovering the Role of Soy Protein in Health (St. Louis: Protein Technologies International, 1999).

Soy Stats 1999: A Reference Guide to Important Soybean Facts and Figures (St. Louis: American Soybean Association, 1999).

2000 Heart and Stroke Statistical Update (Dallas: American Heart Association, 1999).

Wellness Letter 16 (February 2000), University of California, Berkeley.

Your Guide to Soy and the Basic Food Groups (Columbus: Ohio Soybean Council, 1998).

American Academy of Allergy, Asthma, and Immunology Web site (www.aaaai.org).

American Diabetes Web site (www.diabetes.org).

National Osteoporosis Foundation Web site (www.nof.org).

North American Menopause Society Web site (www.menopause.org).

Resources

HEALTH ORGANIZATIONS

American Heart Association
7272 Greenville Ave.
Dallas, TX 75231
800-AHA-USA1
www.americanheart.org

American Cancer Society
1599 Clifton Rd. NE
Atlanta, GA 30329
800-ACS-2345
www.cancer.org

Resources

North American Menopause Society
P.O. Box 94527
Cleveland, OH 44101
800-774-5342
www.menopause.org

National Osteoporosis Foundation
1232 22nd St. N.W.
Washington, D.C. 20037-1292
202-223-2226
www.nof.org

American Diabetes Association
1701 North Beauregard St.
Alexandria, VA 22311
800-342-2383
www.diabetes.org

American Academy of Allergy, Asthma, and Immunology
611 East Wells St.
Milwaukee, WI 53202
800-822-2762
www.aaaai.org

WHERE TO FIND SOY PRODUCTS

www.soyfoods.com

ANSWERS TO QUESTIONS ABOUT SOY AND HEALTH

www.ag.uiuc.edu/~stratsoy/expert/askhealth.html

Glossary

Amino acids   The building blocks of protein. Of the twenty essential amino acids needed to build protein, eleven are naturally produced by the body. The remaining nine amino acids must be supplied by the diet.

Angiogenesis   The process by which new blood vessels develop.

Antioxidant   Beneficial substance found in foods that helps prevent damage to cells.

Atherosclerosis   The thickening of the artery walls with fat deposits, causing narrowing of the arteries that can lead to heart disease or heart attack.

Bone resorption   The breaking down, or loss, of bone tissue.

Calcium   A mineral necessary for building bones and teeth. Also essential for other body functions. The recommended daily allowance for calcium is one thousand milligrams for adults.

Cholesterol   A fat-soluble substance used in the body's metabolism. Found in animal fat and oils, cholesterol contributes to clogging of the arteries, which is a risk factor for heart attacks.

Edamame   Sweet green soybeans that have been harvested before reaching full maturity.

Epidemiological studies
Research studies in which data about human populations is analyzed to determine factors that may influence disease rates.

ERT
Estrogen replacement therapy, a treatment available to women experiencing symptoms of menopause.

Fat
An essential substance in the body that helps deliver and absorb fat-soluble vitamins like A, D, E, and K.

FDA
Food and Drug Administration.

Fermentation
A chemical process in which complex organic compounds break down into simpler substances, especially the conversion of sugar to carbon dioxide and alcohol by yeast.

Genistein
One type of plant chemical studied by

soy researchers that may have potential health benefits.

Grams A metric unit of measurement often used on food labels.

HDL High-density lipoprotein. Often referred to as the "good" cholesterol because it helps reduce and eliminate excess cholesterol in the bloodstream.

HRT Hormone replacement therapy, a treatment available to women experiencing symptoms of menopause.

HVP Hydrolyzed vegetable protein, a substance used by food manufacturers to flavor packaged foods.

In vitro Literally, "in glass." Studies done in vitro are conducted by mixing substances in test tubes or other containers. For example, researchers might add substances from soy to cancer cells to see if the substances have an effect on the growth or proliferation of those cells.

In vivo   Studies conducted in vivo use animals and/or humans. During such studies researchers can test how a disease process in the body is affected by the addition of another substance, like soy.

Isoflavones   Plant chemicals that researchers believe may provide important health benefits.

LDL   Low-density lipoprotein. Often referred to as the "bad" cholesterol because it leaves cholesterol deposits in the bloodstream, which increases heart-disease risk.

Legumes   Plants like beans and peas that grow their seeds in a pod.

Metastasis   The spread of cancerous cells throughout the body.

Monounsaturated fat The healthiest fat because it does not increase cholesterol levels. Sources of monounsaturated fats include olives, avocados, and some nuts.

Natto   Made from fermented soybeans, with a sticky, pasty texture. In Asian countries natto is eaten as a breakfast and as a dinner food. Natto is used as a topping for rice and added to vegetable dishes and miso soup.

Okara   A flaky by-product of soy milk, used in some packaged foods as a fiber additive.

Glossary

Omega-3 fatty acids   Essential fatty acids that benefit the heart and brain.

Polyunsaturated fat   Found in sunflower, safflower, and soybean oil, and healthier than saturated fat. Unfortunately, when polyunsaturated fats are chemically altered to make other products like margarine, they are just as unhealthy as saturated fats.

Protein   Necessary for all cells, protein builds and repairs body tissues.

Saturated fat   Found in animal protein like meat and cheese; remains solid at room temperature. Also promotes cholesterol production in the body and clogs arteries, increasing heart-disease risk.

Soy meat alternatives   "Meat" made out of soy, tofu, or other soy-based products.

Soy protein isolate

The most refined soy product, soy protein isolate is more than 90 percent soy protein, with the fiber removed. It is mainly used by food manufacturers as an ingredient in packaged soups and sauces and in other packaged foods.

Textured soy protein (TSP)

Textured soy protein, also called textured vegetable protein (TVP); made from soy flour and used as a meat extender or replacer and added to processed foods by the food industry.

Triglycerides

The primary type of fat found in foods, used by the body to produce body fat and lipoproteins (that is, cholesterol).

TSP

See textured soy protein.

TVP

See textured soy protein.

Yuba   A popular soy food in China and Japan made from the "skin" that forms on the surface of heated soy milk as it cools.

Index

INDEX

Index

INDEX

Index

INDEX

Index

INDEX

Index

INDEX